Angels Cleopatra and Psychosis

A drug drenched rock'n'roll ride through mental health!

Michael Black

Michael Black

All rights reserved, no part of this publication may be reproduced by any means, electronic, mechanical photocopying, documentary, film or in any other format without prior written permission of the publisher.

Published by
Chipmunkapublishing
PO Box 6872
Brentwood
Essex CM13 1ZT
United Kingdom

http://www.chipmunkapublishing.com

Copyright © Michael Black 2009
Cover Image © Simon Richardson

Chipmunkapublishing gratefully acknowledges the support of Arts Council England.

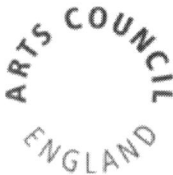

Supported by Macclesfield Mind

"What I've been waiting for!! Thought provoking, humorous, thrilling, magical……… Michael takes you on the ride of your life through mental health. Should be mandatory reading for all "professionals"!!"
Jayne Phillips, Macclesfield **Mind**

Michael Black

FRONTISPIECE

To the memory of Nigel Bailey

Angels, Cleopatra And Psychosis represents five chapters from a larger book I have been writing for the last four years called *Stealing Heaven From God* that will now never see the light of day. It was an attempt to explain in a fully documentary way my psychiatric history since it started in 1993 from my own, not a psychiatrist's, perspective, and at the point where it reached 750 pages with clearly at least another 250 to go, I decided to abandon it. I don't particularly enjoy writing books, I like writing scripts, and I had ceased to enjoy writing it completely. Further, I decided that it was quite simply too long to ever find a publisher. *Stealing Heaven From God* has also been wiped from my computer, and exists only on two CD-ROMs, both stored in secret locations that no one will ever find but me. *Stealing Heaven From God* was also too personally revealing I decided. *Angels, Cleopatra And Psychosis* is not, and I stand by every word. But Nigel Bailey my CPN first encouraged me to write about my spiritual experiences and life within the mental health world, so I dedicate *Angels, Cleopatra And Psychosis* to his memory.

In reducing *Stealing Heaven From God* to these five chapters, a completely coherent narrative of events has of course been lost, but I have decided that doesn't matter. What does is the power and extraordinary nature of the spiritual experiences I have been through, and they remain. The five chapters all open with italicised explanations of their context, and are also contextualised by the *Intro*, the *Interlude*, and the *Outro*.

This is not an academic book, it is essentially a book of autobiographical short stories, and that is another reason I have decided to publish. What is currently written on the subject of spirituality and mental health I find highly inadequate. I refer here to books such as *Psychosis And Spirituality* (ed. Isabel Clarke) and *Spirituality And Mental Health Care* (John Swinton), both published in 2001, and both boringly academic and lacking in real life examples. I have never met a mental hospital patient who would understand either of them!

Thank you.

Michael Black, Macclesfield, August 2007

Angels, Cleopatra and Psychosis

Special thanks to Jayne Phillips of Macclesfield Mind for reading my full psychiatric notes (which run to more than a 1000 pages!), and much more.

Special thanks also to Dr. Tim Lustig and Sharon Boulton for reading the full manuscript version of *Stealing Heaven From God*. Their help has been invaluable. As Ivan Turgenev once said, "I write to gain the respect of people I respect", and I write for them.

Michael Black

Intro

In the October of 1989, my stage play, *Pure Walking Evil* (see my website at www.mwblack.co.uk) opened on the London Fringe at the Old Red Lion theatre to critical acclaim. During the run of the play, the Berlin Wall was torn down by the oppressed citizens of East Berlin. The play concerns the Nazi Minister for Propaganda, Dr. Josef Goebbels interning the Lutheran priest Pastor Martin Niemöller before and during the Second World War 1939-45, and was seen by a director from the National Theatre of Romania, who immediately said he wanted to do the play as well.

That year of 1989 there were revolutions all over Eastern Europe, the Romanian one happening over the Christmas and New Year of 1989/90 after riots erupted in the city of Timisoara over the Securitate secret police arrest of one Pastor Tokes. This was actually the last of the European revolutions of that period, and when the Ceaucescus were shot, Communism was dead too. To the world it was clear that the Soviet leader Mikhail Gorbachev's attempts at reforming Communism from within, increasingly instigated since 1985, had failed. The Cold War was over and the West had won.

Pure Walking Evil opened at the National Theatre of Romania in Timisoara the following Autumn of 1990, before touring and then transferring to the capital Bucharest, the first international new play to be performed in Romania since the revolution itself. Revolutions fascinate me, the French and Russian ones having obsessed my youthful mind for many years, and

Michael Black

here I was in the middle of new one! What a very excited young man I was sitting in the audience on the first night! This was my first experience of performance on a main stage anywhere in the world, and at the end of the first performance the play got a standing ovation. The for so long oppressed Romanians had never seen anything like it, and neither had I. After the performance there was a big press conference, and I was centre stage. The TV lights came on, the press cameras flashed. "This is European theatre" I said. "A play written about German events by an Englishman and performed by Romanians". Germany was by this time a unified country, and I proceeded to give a speech about the possible eastern enlargement of the European Union, an institution I profoundly believe in. I said that "you never know, but in ten years time, Romania might be a member of the EU itself". Everyone laughed at me, but I repeated my point, and OK I was wrong. It didn't take Romania ten years to join the EU, it has taken them sixteen. But nevertheless, that night in Timisoara will remain with me for the rest of my life. I had seen my theatre work performed on a national main stage, albeit not my own, and I knew it had worked. I kept talking. The cameras still flashed, the TV lights were still on and the journalists were still taking notes. That night in Timisoara I felt like a superstar.

Also in 1990, I finally received my doctor of philosophy degree from Cambridge University in English Literature for a thesis on the South African writer Alan Paton. The composition of *Pure Walking Evil* and my doctorate had occupied my mind together for six years together in total, and now I was finally harvesting the fruits of my extensive labours.

Angels, Cleopatra and Psychosis

Discussing the future with Sharon my girlfriend on the lawn of my garden flat in London that summer the future seemed remarkably simple. Get a teaching job in a university, continue writing successful stage plays, get married and start having babies. On the strength of such expectations Sharon and I were married in February of 1991, and our son Robert was born later that year. I felt I had, or would soon have it all.

But then life can kick you in the teeth, can't it? After the birth of Robert, I soon found out that the good times were over, big style! The job I wanted in a university simply wasn't there in those educationally ravaged Thatcherite times. And writing successful follow up plays to *Pure Walking Evil* and raising the money to do them with a new wife and child around the house proved much more difficult than I had ever imagined. Suddenly I was writing with responsibilities in mind, whereas before I had been writing with a free mind. Two different things. I was the man of the house and new father, but, despite an Arts Council bursary to write a new play about Beethoven, heading for the dole queue. £5000 doesn't go very far on a mortgage, wife and child...

I hated unemployment, and I hated the (technically legal) deception of it all that I continued to work as a writer during this period. And I hated the endless grind of applying for university jobs that it had become all too apparent I would not get. No one wanted an expert on South African literature, everyone wanted the boringly canonical Ph.Ds on Shakespeare, Byron, Henry James, Dickens and so on. The academic system will forever repeat itself! Further, nothing puts strain on a relationship like a first baby, life for both partners changes completely, and I was also working from home. My relationship with Sharon became daily more fractious and claustrophobic, and I resorted to drinking too much in pubs I didn't even like just to get away from it all. Everything just kept going from bad to worse, and even my biggest hero Kenny Dalglish let me down, walking out on his job as manager of Liverpool FC in February 1991.

They say that being lionised by premature success is one of the worst things that can happen to a young writer, and after the above described experiences, looking at it all seventeen years down the line, I think that is true. Both in terms of academia and theatre I had expectations of what the future had in store for me that were totally out of line with reality. Academics don't really take theatre or playwrights seriously anyway, and I was trying to be both. I still insist there's nothing wrong with the attempted combination, but realistically I should have seen that the deal was never going to come off, and thought of another plan.

I could go on with this story but I'm not going to. Suffice to say that the saying "if something can go wrong it will go wrong" proved true of my life from 1990 to 1995. Sharon and I were divorced that year, and by then I hadn't had a play production for five years either. I spent five years going first quietly and after that rather loudly mad. Mad people live in mental hospitals, and that's where I was soon enough as well.

Angels, Cleopatra and Psychosis

You don't think this is all that funny do you? But now, writing in the summer of 2007, in many ways I do. So after a total of fourteen years in and out of psychiatric wards, after four different psychiatric diagnoses (hypomania, schizophrenia, manic depression and schizoaffective disorder), and after endless arguments with psychiatrists and psychiatric nurses, I'm finally going to tell the story my way, and not theirs.

It's all true, I swear it, I've had an extraordinary time, and here goes.

Michael Black

A Meeting With Michelangelo
Now there I go again with my crystal visions
I keep my visions to myself
Fleetwood Mac, *Dreams*

I first met Michelangelo on Newark railway station in the June of 1993. I was already in a strange mood, feeling very light headed, but also very intellectually energetic. Emotionally though, I was fragile. By this time, Sharon and I were living separate lives in Hertfordshire and York respectively, and I had caught a train from Glasgow where I had seen relatives to go back down south. The canteen on the train was closed and I had an open ticket for any train, so I decided to get off at Newark to get a cup of tea before getting back on the next train going to London. Simple. The platform was empty and there he was, an invisible shining spirit of handsome male strength with cascading hair, a living transparent yet almost translucent force field of energy and life-after-death. He looked like his own statue of David. I knew immediately it was Michelangelo, there was no need of words or other kinds of confirmation, just as I would know who all the other spirits were when I later met their spirits too. This being was a being like no other I had ever met and doubtless ever will.

And it's all a lot stranger than that. On the train from Glasgow to Newark, looking out of the window for no reason, it had started raining on one side of the train, and was still sunny on the other. A rainbow arched the skies. The heavy rain clouds parted in unison and three female angels winged their way across the skies, all with trumpets, simply radiating

Angels, Cleopatra and Psychosis

triumph. But the triumph of what I thought? Two strong naked male figures appeared, each with their index fingers pointing at the other, but the radiance of the sun soon blinded them from my view as the angels continued to traverse the Heavens and the dance of light on the rolling clouds travelled on. The sky was turning into the Sistine Chapel ceiling, except it was a moving, dynamic version, unrestrained by the static dimensions of a simple fresco or painting. And I know all this to be a moving rendition of the Sistine Chapel ceiling now, but I swear blind that at the time I knew very little about perhaps Michelangelo's most famous work of art at all.

In fact to this day I know very little about the historical Michelangelo, and as the years of knowing his spirit have gone on, I've made it my business not to find out. Why bother? When his spirit first appeared before me that June afternoon, you could say I hardly knew him from Adam.

Newark railway station that afternoon was thankfully very quiet, and I spent four hours speaking with Michelangelo, completely losing track of time in the process. At first I talked out loud to him, but then realised I only had to think to him, and he would think back. His form was transparent and yet radiant with energy to me, and the occasional station porter who passed by obviously saw nothing at all. The porter's problem I suppose.

This of course as I was to discover as the years went by is one of the major problems with spirits, but it is also one of their chief virtues. They only appear to the people they want to appear to, and everyone else is unconscious of their presence at all, but I hadn't worked that out yet on Newark railway station, not least because I'd never met a spirit before in my life, and what's more, it didn't take me long to work out that this was a very powerful one who must have a significant reason for having turned up at all.

Why me? Well, that's pretty much what I asked Michelangelo all afternoon, and yes, I did question my own sanity very deeply indeed. In fact, I was at one point fairly convinced I had completely lost my mind, and it was only Michelangelo's constant insistence to the contrary that convinced me I hadn't. He knew everything about me, and said he'd been watching me for years, and given what he knew, it was fairly obvious that he was telling the truth. Everyone has done things they are ashamed of after all and Michelangelo knew all about those things too, this at first being a very frightening experience because I was briefly convinced he was only here to banish me to Hell.

I said I didn't believe in Hell.
"Neither do I Michael", said Michelangelo. "But unfortunately, it does exist"

I said I didn't believe in God.
"Neither do I Michael", said Michelangelo. "But unfortunately, He exists too".

I said I didn't believe in Heaven.
"You will do Michael", said Michelangelo.

Angels, Cleopatra and Psychosis

I said I didn't want to die. Michelangelo assured me that wasn't on the cards.

I walked up and down the station platform, turned round and round, checked the time, walked out into the station car park and came back again. Michelangelo was still there. *Had I gone completely mad in one train journey alone?* I decided to ask Michelangelo some questions. If he knew the answers to questions I didn't know the answer to, then he had to be real. Simple as that.

Michelangelo was very patient with me. I know very little in fact about high renaissance art, so I started with the basics, and obviously, these biographical facts I have checked since, in fact I checked them as soon as I could find a public library, but that was to be longer than I expected, as you will discover.

"What year were you born?", I said.
"1475", said Michelangelo. "But that doesn't matter".
"Where?".
"Caprese. But I grew up in Florence".
"What's the name of your father? I'm sorry. I have to know".

I could see Michelangelo was getting bored, and as I would come to discover, his boredom threshold is incredibly low. He doesn't hang around for no reason for anyone.

"Please, I need to know".

"Lodovico", said Michelangelo. "Michael, calm down. You are not mad and I am really here. Spirit worlds exist, that's all, and I'm the strongest spirit there is".

For some reason I said I had to get the next train to London, but I had no intention of going anywhere anyway.

"Don't get on a train Michael. Stay here. In fact, you've got no choice. I'm sorry, but it's true".
"Why me?", I said, suddenly feeling desperately alone and rather lost.
"Because you've got perfect timing Michael", said Michelangelo. "You get things right when it matters".
"I've seen visions of angels in the sky today", I said. "And now you. What's going on?"

At this point, I have to repeat that I had never seen a reproduction of the Sistine Chapel Ceiling in my life. And my lack of knowledge about high renaissance art has already been mentioned as well.

"What do you mean I've got perfect timing? About what?".
"About everything that matters Michael. I've been watching you".

It was news to me. Well, it would be, wouldn't it? And what did he mean he'd been watching me?

Angels, Cleopatra and Psychosis

"In bed with girls for example?", I asked somewhat indignantly.

"Generally speaking no Michael", said Michelangelo, "I know how to mind my own business. But I did watch you with Catherine two days ago, and I thought you were very gentle with her. Well done".

"Well done! It's none of your business. Now listen here!"

"It doesn't matter Michael. Come on…". Michelangelo started laughing.

A married man, I had slept with Catherine, a very beautiful twenty year old I had once previously taught for A Levels two days before exactly as Michelangelo said, and I felt awful about it. My marriage was falling apart, I knew it, and it was one of the reasons I was in such a strange mood. Marriage vows were important to me, and I'd never broken them before.

Further, I still didn't really trust the spirit of Michelangelo, still less the moving rendition of the Sistine Chapel ceiling, but at the same time, these were definitely the most real experiences I had ever had in my life. I was screwing up I suppose, but then my ability to differentiate between spirit reality and what most normal people call reality most of the time wasn't very good in 1993, which I think given my lack of practice is understandable. Looking back at it all, everything that followed was totally predictable and inevitable. And I certainly don't blame the spirit of Michelangelo! Eventually, I decided for some reason the best bet was a taxi, and walked to the station taxi rank. The spirit of Michelangelo followed me. I found a taxi, in fact the only one there. It must have been about five o'clock in the afternoon.

"Take me to the Sistine Chapel", I said.
"Where?", said the taxi driver.
"I don't know", I said. I suddenly realised I didn't know where the Sistine Chapel was. Somewhere in Italy certainly, but where? I guessed "Florence".
"Florence! I don't go that far", said the taxi driver.

We had an argument, but it was going nowhere. I had no money, I had no credit cards, so Florence was out of the question anyway. Further, the taxi driver obviously thought I was mad.

"Listen mate, you've been hanging round this station for four hours going nowhere. Something's wrong with you".

But I persevered, determined to go somewhere. *But where?* The answer to everything obviously lay in the vision in the sky of the Sistine Chapel ceiling I had seen. But you can't get a taxi driver to take you to see that.

I suddenly realised I had left my travel bag, my only possession at the time, on the station platform and went to retrieve it. Luckily, it was still there and hadn't been stolen. Michelangelo followed me.

"Michael. Stick with the taxi driver. He'll take you somewhere eventually, and it's bound to be the right place".

Angels, Cleopatra and Psychosis

"I'm totally lost", I said.

"I know", said Michelangelo, for the first time putting his spirit hand around my left wrist.

It felt like an invisible magic bracelet of warmth and love. It was.

"Stick with the taxi driver?"

"Stick with the taxi driver. And wherever you end up, believe me I'll be there too".

So with that I walked back to the taxi driver complete with my travel bag, and, confident the spirit of Michelangelo was beside me, I opened the taxi passenger door and sat down on the car seat.

"Take me to the Sistine Chapel. Florence. Italy".

"Listen mate. Get out of my car. I'm taking you nowhere".

"The Sistine Chapel please".

"Get out of my fucking car!".

"I'm not moving, and I'll pay".

I had no idea how I would pay by the way anyway, but Michelangelo was sitting on the back seat by now and had his hand on my shoulder. I pressed my case.

"Take me to the Sistine Chapel!"

"Alright mate", said the taxi driver. "Calm down. I'll take you wherever you want".

I think by this point the taxi driver was worried I might have started a fight and won it, which I had no intention of doing, but I seemed to be getting my way, didn't I? Maybe the taxi driver thought I might beat him up and steal his motor. I don't know. But needless to say he didn't take me to the Sistine Chapel. He took me straight to Newark Police station instead.

"Why are we stopping here?", I said, with a first sense of foreboding.
"Hang on mate", said the taxi driver. "Just stay there OK?"

Michelangelo's invisible hand was still on my shoulder, but it didn't stop me feeling frightened. I was in trouble, and I was beginning to realise it. I stayed in the car, and two policemen came out of the station to question me. Now, I don't play policemen for a sense of humour, and it was obvious to me that insisting on being taken to the Sistine Chapel was not the right thing to say any more, so I didn't.

I can't exactly remember what happened next, but suffice to say I ended up being questioned in the police station cells alone (well, alone except for the spirit of Michelangelo). It was cold and dark, and the room had nothing I remember in it at all, not even a chair, except for an interview tape recorder on a table, which wasn't used, shame to say, because I would love to hear an interview of the following conversation now, which even I can only partly recall. The walls were covered in disgusting anally orientated graffiti, and I remember being thirsty and in need of a drink which was never offered. I was frightened and disorientated, but I wasn't panicking, possibly because I knew Michelangelo was still with me, and just leaning against a wall saying nothing. But I knew somewhere he was having a good time.

The first policeman to interview me almost immediately told me he used to be a Roman Catholic priest.

"What a surprise!", said Michelangelo. "We are definitely in the right place Michael". He started laughing.

I'd said very little up to this point, and the policeman searched my filofax for phone numbers. I decided to make two phone calls (or did he make them for me?), and realised both were mistakes almost immediately. I rang my mother and then put the phone down when she answered. The policeman had spoken to her first I think, and all I remember is her panicked tone as she shouted "Michael!" as she realised where I was. And then I rang my wife, Sharon, and explaining I was in a police station, then asked her to ring Catherine, whom she knew, just to make sure Catherine was alright. Guilt I suppose, and one hell of a request looking back on it, but for some reason I was worried about Catherine's safety. I suddenly realised I was in great danger, and those around me might be too. Only Michelangelo was calm and assured.

"I've been in worse situations than this Michael, believe me".

Michael Black

The Roman Catholic priest turned policeman told me he thought I was very ill. "Yes I am ill" said a voice I've never heard before coming out of my own mouth, but definitely not mine. I fought the impostor voice immediately without knowing who it was, but I knew if I didn't fight it now, it would take me over forever. "I am not ill" I said to the policeman very definitely and with great considered control. It was a battle, but I won it.

"You'll be alright after that delivery Michael", said Michelangelo. "Believe me, you'll be fine".

But I have to confess I didn't feel it at the time. I was scared, and I knew I was in big trouble. I was locked in a police cell without having committed any crime or done anything remotely violent, and it was obvious they weren't going to let me go.

"Welcome to the revolution", said Michelangelo.

I got annoyed with him at this point, I felt tricked by the moving Sistine Chapel sky, and yes, of course, talking to the spirit of Michelangelo again, I was still very deeply questioning my own sanity. But this was a police cell, there was graffiti on the walls, I *was* talking to policemen and so on. It was obvious to me I knew where I was, I could remember how I had ended up there and so on. I decided again I was *not* losing my marbles, and that the spirit of Michelangelo was the only being around with any real intelligence and knowledge.

Angels, Cleopatra and Psychosis

I noticed the police cell door was not locked and opened it and walked down the corridor. All the other cells were empty, but they were full of graffiti too and the whole place smelt of urine. A very nice policeman with a Nottinghamshire accent stopped me and very caringly suggested I go back to the cell I had originally been put in. I agreed. Well, there was nowhere better, was there?

"Don't worry", said the policeman. "There are some people coming to see you, that's all".

But I was worried wasn't I? I was bound to be, more than… And I didn't need to ask Michelangelo who those people were going to be. It was obvious to me that I was about to be interviewed by a psychiatrist. And various cohorts. The nightmare was about to begin.

"Michael", said Michelangelo. "You know what is coming next, and we have to talk quickly. This isn't going to be easy for any of us…"

"Who do you mean? Any of us?", I asked.

"It can wait. But we're not going to lose, believe me. Never forget that. But you have to know a few things quickly".

"Like what?".

"Like the Sistine Chapel ceiling Michael", Michelangelo said laughing, "is not in Florence! It's the Pope's chapel in the Vatican Michael".

"Really?". I was dumbfounded, and I knew this was important.

"Really. The Vatican Michael, and believe me, that place is the heart of all darkness. I lived and worked there – against my will Michael – and I should know".

"But you did paint it?".

"Of course I painted it. No other painter could possibly have painted it! But the true story has never been told, so listen carefully…"

I was listening as I had never listened to anyone before in my life, but then it happened, and somehow I saw it coming just in time. The invisible hand of an invisible but incredibly powerful Cardinal reached straight inside my body, and started to squeeze the life out of my heart. I couldn't breathe, my heart was no longer beating!

"NO!" I screamed. "NO! No, no no…"

My heart started to beat again slightly, the Cardinal was losing, and he knew it. "No. No. No". Pause for breathe. "No". Pause for another one. "No". I repeated these words to the increasing rhythm of my heartbeat as it returned. "No. No. No". As simple as that.

I had survived death for the first time, and I knew it.

"Michael", said Michelangelo, "you are in business".

But I didn't feel in business at all. I felt utterly terrified and I just didn't know what was going on any more. The very nice policeman came in the cell and asked me if I was alright. I said I was. "Yes, fine mate, forget it". "Something troubling you?". "No, not at all". That sort of thing.

"There's some people to see you now Michael".
"Right", I said. What else was I supposed to say?

I breathed very deeply and looked at Michelangelo, still leaning against the wall in a corner of the cell. Never a spirit of unnecessary reassurance, he didn't say anything, he just kept leaning there.

"You got me into this", I said.
"I know", he replied. "Inevitable".

The nice policemen brought in four chairs. And three people arrived shortly afterwards, one woman and two men I think, but I only remember the woman now, and I can't remember her name. She transpired to be the psychiatrist. I decided immediately I wasn't going to be humble or careful or even particularly respectful, although I also had no intention of being openly rude. But after the day I'd had – Sistine Chapel ceiling skies, the spirit of Michelangelo, an invisible Cardinal trying to kill me – there was no point pretending everything was normal, was there?

The psychiatrist was careful in her questioning of me, but I can't remember what the questions were. It was obvious she thought I was very ill. Well, she'd probably got a story from a Roman Catholic priest turned policeman that I'd got in a taxi and started a row about going to the Sistine Chapel, hadn't she? *What was the point acting sane at all?, and what was sanity anyway?* She asked me who I was, where I was born and so on, so I said my name, and Liverpool in 1962, which it suddenly occurred to me was the same year that the Beatles made it big. A strange coincidence I thought (it had never occurred to me in my life before), and I pondered the meaning of synchronicity once again, a subject that has long fascinated me. You can plan your life as much as you like, but sometimes things just happen at the right or wrong time, or just don't happen at all, and there is frequently more wisdom to be divined through that than in anything else. And of course, *Synchronicity* is the title of the last Police album as well…

I was still pondering the year 1962 and ran a few Beatles lyrics through my head, thinking of singing a few to her. *Well, why not?* And I certainly was in no mood to have my personality analysed by someone I didn't even know. *That was definitely not going to happen!* And then it became absolutely apparent what I should do. The Cardinal's invisible hand in mind, I decided to launch into a rendition of Bob Dylan's *Highway 61 Revisited*, first verse only.

God said to Abraham "kill me a son"
Abe said "God you must be putting me on"
God said "no", Abe said "what?"
God said "you can do what you want Abe but
The next time you see me coming you better run"
And Abe said "where d'you want the killing done?"
And God said "out on Highway 61!"

Angels, Cleopatra and Psychosis

And then I stopped. There was silence, and the two other people with the psychiatrist started writing copious notes. I wonder what about to this day, but they certainly weren't transcribing Bob Dylan lyrics were they? More pity for them.

Everything was apparent to me now! Don't ask me why Dylan set his song on Highway 61, but the story of God testing the loyalty of Abraham – or Ibrahim – by asking him to kill his son and only calling the whole cruel game off when Abraham is about to literally put the knife in, is common to Judaism, Christianity and Islam after all. I mean, what is that story about, and how can anybody – or Anybody – be so cruel!? We all suffer the meanings of that story to this day if you see what I mean, and the true meaning of it is loud and clear.

"God's a bastard", I said. "A cruel sadistic bastard".

"Really?". That's all the psychiatrist said in response! But I was rocking. *"God is a cruel sadistic bastard, and he sticks the knife into people only to test your loyalty and do it again the next time, and there's no end it!"*

"And God's a rapist too!", I shouted.

Revelations like this make you angry, and I have never been so angry in my life. I was thinking of Zeus raping Leda and Europa, it all made sense, but the psychiatrist didn't seem to agree, and neither was I given chance to explain.

Yes, it was obvious the psychiatrist thought I was barking mad, but I didn't care. *"God is a bastard!"*, that was the point of the day I'd had, and after the Cardinal's failed attempt to kill me, what did I have to fear saying it? The problem afflicting the planet was clearly God, and I intended to do something about it. *My life's mission was clear!* And Michelangelo was still leaning against a wall in the corner (although obviously the psychiatrist and her two cohorts didn't know this), so what did I care what some two dime shrink thought of my lyric singing? It all made sense to me, and that was the most important thing. I wanted to ask Michelangelo just how he'd arranged for a moving rendition of the Sistine Chapel ceiling to vault the skies, but decided against it. Talking to what to a psychiatrist would appear to be an empty wall was obviously not a good idea at this point, and besides, I doubted Michelangelo would tell me the answer. There's a time and a place for everything, and this wasn't it.

It was fairly apparent to me by this point that the next stop was a mental hospital, but *c'est la vie*. The nightmare of my life was about to begin, but I was determined to enter the nightmare on my own terms. And I certainly wasn't going anywhere by force. So I said so, and the rest of the interview was conducted in very polite terms. The psychiatrist started looking for angles. Would I be prepared to be taken somewhere in a police car? "No", I said, "most definitely not, I'd prefer a carriage". Michelangelo started laughing hysterically, so I carried on. "Why a carriage?", said the psychiatrist. "Well, I like to travel in a civilised and

Angels, Cleopatra and Psychosis

leisurely manner",I replied. The psychiatrist was lost for words.

I mean, and I've thought it many times since, just what are you supposed to say to these people, and where on earth is their sense of humour?! They ask you the most mundane, stupid and BORING questions, and somehow you are the one in the dock with the sanity problem! *"How are you today? How has your week gone? You are seeming much more stable today"*. I mean, seriously, come on! *How do you reply to questions like that?* And a psychiatrist's definition of sanity by the way is always dull incuriosity, being a well adjusted clone of the system, but I hadn't worked that out in the police station I was still sitting in in June 1993.

What I had worked out is that a carriage was out of the question. So without narrating the police station scene any longer – and I can't remember any more anyway – suffice to say that I had to back down on a carriage and settle for an ambulance, but that's definitely one up from a police car in my book, so I entered the nightmare winning, and Michelangelo came too, so what did I care. The ambulance took me to a mental hospital in Mansfield, and instead of policemen inside it, like I'd committed some crime, I remember two paramedics inside it instead, and they didn't say very much, but they were very nice to me and in no way threatening.

I entered the Mansfield mental hospital – I forget the name of it – in a very strange but elated mood. The whole thing seemed hilarious to me, I mean, just what had I supposedly done wrong?, and like how come I was the only person that day to have seen Michelangelo's Sistine Chapel traverse the skies? It had been clearly visible, but it was also obvious to me that you would have had to have been looking at the sky at the time, and most people go through life with their heads down at a desk all day. Further, maybe the Sistine Chapel sky was only *there if you had the imagination to see it!* You know what I mean?

Anyway, the mental hospital wasn't pleasant, but it wasn't some dark dungeon either, it was somewhere between the two, as they almost always are.

But there the story takes its first of many dark turns. I was elated, I was rocking, I was hanging around with the spirit of Michelangelo who was still right by my side. *What could these people do to harm me?* But I didn't know anything about mental hospitals yet did I? If I had met Michelangelo that day, who on earth was I about to meet next? The answer was obvious to me, and it had to be Leonardo da Vinci! I didn't know much about high Renaissance art, but even I could work that one out. Leonardo had to follow on from Michelangelo, and Michelangelo wasn't saying anything to tell me I was wrong, so I went for it. Running down the ward corridor determined to run through the door at the end of it, "Michelangelo is here" I shouted, "and Leonardo must be around somewhere too. Let's go and find him! Come on! Let's go!".

I was immediately surrounded by six male nurses and pinned to the floor. There was a struggle, but I gave up struggling when it was obvious that to struggle any more risked them physically harming me. They pulled my trousers down and shoved a needle full of some chemical up my arse.

Michelangelo just watched. I guess he'd seen it all before.

That's all I remember.

The next day, I woke up in a bed on the ward feeling OK, and suffering from a risen Christ delusion, my first. But I quickly worked out I could not possibly be the risen Christ, not least because I didn't believe in Him anyway, and figured it must be a trick of the invisible Cardinal.

"Correct", said Michelangelo, sitting at the end of my bed.
"Where am I?".
"In a mental hospital in Mansfield. Do you remember yesterday?".
"Like a dream", I said.

I was still rocking inside, but I had calmed down to the world and worked out that I was incarcerated without committing any crime. *What to do next?* I decided to get to know the layout of the ward, and soon found out it had most of the usual features these places always do have. There was a TV lounge full of cigarette smoke, a nurses office which almost always seem to have more nurses in them than are out on the ward, a desk with something like "Nurse Base Area" written on it, and so on. I was sleeping in an open dormitory of perhaps six beds, but there were some individual bedrooms at the far end of the ward with some very strange people inside them indeed. These people were on fifteen minute observations, or "15 minute obs" as they are called, and each of these rooms had a nurse permanently outside them. I decided I didn't want to get to know the people inside.

I also decided to stick around the other end of the ward in the TV lounge and smoked a few cigarettes, but even I couldn't take that much cigarette smoke hanging around in the air, and the room was full of gormless people just watching TV for no good reason at all. This is the average day to day reality of the average mental ward, and it is incredibly tedious, and it can go on for months at a time, interspersed only by the odd deranged psychotic kicking off occasionally and trashing the lighting system or the TV or whatever. But that never happened in Mansfield. In fact, nothing much happened in Mansfield at all in one sense, but it was all very significant in another, simply because it was my first introduction to mental hospitals. Welcome to the real world, if you see what I mean.

It was apparent to me there was very little intelligence or life about anywhere, although at the time I didn't realise how debilitating psychiatric drugs can be on those unfortunate enough to have to take them. Some of them do turn you into a zombie, simple as that.

I decided to find out exactly what the score was. I talked to the nurses, who told me I had "a long way to go" before I was likely to be let out, which didn't exactly make me feel wonderful, but at the same time I didn't take it too seriously. *Who were these people and just what was their problem?* I found out though that I was on a Section 2, which means I had been detained under the Mental Health Act for 28 days. I now know it actually means by the way for "up to 28 days", but that's not what I was told at the time, and I was determined to get out as fast as possible. *But how?* I started to feel depressed. I was in a mental hospital, I had no immediate way out, my boredom threshold is incredibly low, and 28 days seemed like an eternity. This was a nightmare, there was no question about it, but I knew I had to fight back or spiritually capitulate forever, and I decided the best way of fighting back was playing it cool. Act like you're not concerned. Well, that's what Michelangelo was still doing, so why shouldn't I?

I was told I had to take a drug called Haloperidol, which comes in the form of a pink tablet, and I was also told that if I refused, it would be injected into me forcibly if necessary. So I took it, obviously, wondering at the time if thought power would be enough to resist whatever its effects were, which, obviously, I didn't know yet.

That weekend, concerned relatives converged on me from all parts of the country. Sharon came from Hertfordshire with her sister Brigitte, and my mother came from Wilmslow with her younger sister Pat and her husband Frank, who had travelled all the way from Glasgow. Now I like all these people to this day, but the disconcerting thing was how disconcerted they all were, particularly my mother, who I knew would take the opinion of any psychiatrist far too seriously for her own or my good. My father had been sent to see a psychiatrist just before my parents got divorced in about 1973, and I remember my mother saying then to me that "you have always to assume that these people are at least as bright as you are". Well, I instinctively disagreed with that statement when I was eleven years old, and, after fourteen years in and out of the psychiatric system, I most certainly disagree with it now. Most psychiatrists, and a great many nurses, are stupid. It is as simple as that.

Sharon said only 90% of what I was saying was making sense, but since to me that means a far greater percentage than is usual in most human discourse, I couldn't see what her problem was either. But I did know she was obviously frightened to have a husband in a mental hospital, and it was going to be difficult to get any kind of real relationship back with her from here. Obviously, I didn't tell any one about moving Sistine Chapel ceiling skies or the presence of the spirit of Michelangelo. Then they really would have been concerned, wouldn't they! And my mother would probably have gone straight to a nurse or psychiatrist and spilled the beans so to speak! No thank you.

I was in a very difficult situation.

And then the Haloperidol kicked in. I was walking around the hospital grounds about three days into my incarceration when my spine suddenly twisted backwards with a massive muscle spasm. I couldn't remotely walk, and fell over reeling on the ground. I was in agony.

"Michael!", shouted a nurse, "get up!".

"I can't".
"Get up!".

Michelangelo just watched it all happen. He'd obviously seen it before.

"Get up!".
"I can't".

But I eventually did get up somehow, and made it back to the ward. I realised that mental hospitals are like policemen. You don't play them for laughs. I sat down at the first chair in sight, which happened to be in the nurses' office.

"Get out of here Michael!".
"I can't walk".
"You walked in here! Get out!".

Michelangelo put his hands on his forehead. He'd definitely seen all this before. I made it out of the nurses' office and back to my bed.

"What's going on?", I said to Michelangelo. I was seriously worried.
"It's the drugs Michael. They'll put you on a drug called Procyclidine to stop the side effects as they say about what they call "muscle stiffness", but it won't work. You're in trouble".
"You got me into this".
"I know".
"Then get me out of it".
"I can't. That's your job".
"This is a nightmare".

"That's life".
"You've tricked me".
"In a way, yes. But I had no choice".

And then Michelangelo started fading away in front of my eyes.

"Don't go", I said.
"I'm not going anywhere Michael".
"You are! You're vanishing".
"I'm not. But you're losing your ability to talk with me or know I'm here. It's the drugs Michael. That's what they do to people, and it's probably what they're supposed to do. They stop people talking with spirit worlds. I'm sorry, but you're going to lose contact with me".
"But you'll still be here really?".
"I…".

And after that I lost contact with Michelangelo completely. I was terrified. None of this was remotely funny any more. Singing *Highway 61 Revisited* to a psychiatrist was starting to feel like a seriously big mistake. And I was frightened of the invisible Cardinal too. I might have survived the heart attack attempt, but how many ways was he going to find to torture me now? I didn't know where my protection was any more did I?

The rest is predictable. I was put on Procyclidine to counter the muscle spasm back twisting effects of Haloperidol, and it didn't work. I didn't get the muscle spasms any more, but I started walking around like a zombie. All my natural sense of balance

Angels, Cleopatra and Psychosis

and movement had gone. *And let's get the logic straight right now! If a drug causes your spine to twist backwards, the logical thing is not to give you another drug to stop it happening. The logical thing is to take you off the first drug! Right?* Exactly.

But I was powerless to say that at the time and no one would have listened any way. I was learning the rules of an entirely new world, and I didn't like them at all. But I knew I was going to have to endure them, and I also knew even then that I was not going to give in.

I got a letter from Catherine saying how much she cared for me. It meant a lot at the time, and it was beginning to feel like she was the only person in the world who really did. Everyone else thought I had serious psychiatric problems! I came to the conclusion I had serious problems with psychiatrists. And I was going to have to endure all this for at least 28 days, which, as I have said, seemed like an eternity. But boy, was I going to fight! Somehow, boy, was I going to fight!

I lay on my bed for days trying to think of how. I couldn't think how at all.

There was nothing to do, the whole place was tedious in the extreme, but one day I did make it to the canteen. I tried to be polite and debonair to the canteen lady, but with my natural sense of movement gone, it was extremely difficult.

"Can I have a cup of tea and a scone please".
"Do you pay or does it go on the account?".

Michael Black

"I'm sorry?".
"Are you a doctor here?".

Well, I did have a doctorate from Cambridge University, didn't I? Dr. Michael Black, Ph.D., Cantab.

Was I a doctor? I said I wasn't sure. And it was an interesting question. What did she mean, and had she ever thought about it? Who were the real doctors around here?

And then after about five days they just let me go. I didn't ask any questions. I just packed my bags and got the first train to Hertfordshire to stay with Sharon's parents. I was still on Haloperidol and Procyclidine, but at least I wasn't in a mental hospital any more. In other words, I legged it fast.

Looking back on it now, I had escaped from my first mental hospital in record time, but I had no idea how. And for once in my life, I wasn't asking any questions.

Devil At the Door!

The greatest wile of the Devil is to convince you He doesn't exist.
Charles Baudelaire

A terraced house in north York. By now my marriage was on the rocks. After we were married, Sharon and I had left London for York, hoping to lower our overheads I suppose, and presuming she could find work there as a teacher whilst I looked after our young son Robert and continued to write. I was working on my Beethoven play, and also on my experimental novel *Crossing Out The Emperor*, which is available to this day as a free download from my website www.mwblack.co.uk. But Sharon could not find work, and eventually left for a new teaching job back down south in Welwyn Garden City, taking Robert with her. I was living on my own, but I was quickly to find in many ways I was not. The spirit of Michelangelo turned up again to be with me, and with him came the spirit of Leonardo da Vinci. They explained they had long since put their past differences behind them, and that they were on two missions, one of cosmic significance, the other personal. The long standing one of cosmic significance was to work out how to steal God's power and build a better and more just world in consequence, since God was clearly incapable of doing so after so long in power. The second personal mission, they explained was the rescue of a girl. The girl's name was Romancia, she was long since dead, but her spirit still lived. Unfortunately however, at her death the Devil had trapped her in Hell, where she had been for the past five hundred years. I constantly asked them why *the girl was so important, and Michelangelo eventually explained that Romancia had been Leonardo's one true love and girlfriend. There were tears in Leonardo's eyes as Michelangelo told me…*

The next few hours were terrifying and are hard to describe. Darkness somehow fell almost immediately that day or seemed to, and by the evening I knew I was effectively living in Hell. It was still June in 1994, and the lights in the house still worked of course, but didn't seem to make any difference to how dark it was. So I decided to close all the curtains – I didn't want anyone passing by to look in. The invisible Cardinal's presence was everywhere. I could move around the house, but the spirits of Leonardo da Vinci and Michelangelo were still stuck in my office-bedroom, so I was on my own, with no intention of going outside. Or at least not for now. That, I instinctively felt would only make matters worse.

I had been living and working almost exclusively in my office-bedroom with Leonardo and Michelangelo, and I realised how damp it felt downstairs. The clay tile floor let Hell up through the ground or so it now seemed. The dampness seemed to pull my feet down. I started to wonder how solid the floor was! Could I sink through it?

By 9pm or thereabouts I was effectively trapped downstairs, and the invisible Cardinal challenged me to go back up the stairs and see if Leonardo and Michelangelo could provide any safety. Since I knew they couldn't, I didn't bother. The Cardinal would not have suggested it if it would have helped me, and it was obvious that this battle with the Cardinal was all mine. He challenged me to walk right through him to mount the stairs, blocking my way as he did so, but I didn't bother. What would it have gained me? I would only have to have come downstairs again, since I instinctively knew this would be the scene of the battle.

The Cardinal tells me I had been foolish to listen to Leonardo and Michelangelo. He tells me they know nothing important (they tell me they are my friends and that God is persecuting me to death). Then the Cardinal tells me that this is my last night on earth. I tell the Cardinal I don't believe him, and that if he wants a fight he's got one. I add that if Leonardo and Michelangelo didn't count for anything, they would have been consigned to Hell a long time ago, and that I'll take my own chances. I remember what my illustrious friends have said about the Cardinal's arrogance, and remember that if his heart attack didn't kill me the first time, what was he going to come up with this time?

"Just you wait and see", he says. The Cardinal can obviously read my mind, but I don't care, or try not to.

However, it hardly makes my situation easier. How do I get away from him without him knowing?

"You obviously want a fight, and you've got one", I say. "I am going to survive, and the real battle with you starts here from what I can see".

The Cardinal simply laughs.

"It does indeed", he says, revealing a spiked ball and chain from behind his back.
"Threats won't make me back off" I say, but I'm realising this is going to be some night.

How real is the spiked ball and chain I wonder? Can it physically damage me, or is it some kind of metaphysical trick? I realise that at some point I am probably going to have to find out, and I also realise I have a bottle of red wine in the house and I open it, but I don't drink much. It was going to have to last, and I am going to need a clear head!

"You haven't met the Devil yet", says the Cardinal.
"I'm obviously going to though, aren't I?", I reply.

By now I'm terrified beyond measure, but also feeling incredibly strong and brave. My adrenalin levels must have been through the ceiling! And luckily the CD player was downstairs too with a few CDs, including *Achtung Baby* by U2. I realise that this is partly a challenge about how much darkness I can survive, so let's bring it on, because what could be darker than that?, and I knew some rock'n'roll would help me. I couldn't believe that the Cardinal liked music like this, so I played it loud. *Even Better Than the Real Thing* and *She Moves In Mysterious Ways*.

Henry my Welsh collie-German Shepherd crossed dog was in his basket and I realise he is sitting up and paying attention to everything that is going on. I consider my options, including at some point leaving the house with Henry as my protector, so check to see where my house keys are. They appear to have gone missing, which is highly unusual for me. I always double check where everything is.

The Cardinal laughs.

"Find them now!", he says.

So I determine to.

"What is the trick you play?", I ask, *Ultra Violet* blasting through the CD player. "Baby, baby, light my way…"

The Cardinal comes after me with his spiked ball and chain, and I have no intention to find out whether it is metaphysical or real. I don't want to have my head smashed, so I duck and dive to the rhythms of the music. My first victory!, because I realise my sense of timing is better than the Cardinal's.

"What is the trick you play?", I repeat. "I need to find my house keys, and I'm not backing down".

I suddenly realise what the trick is, and realise the Cardinal can interfere with the workings of your mind without you realising.

"You make me put things in places I won't remember!", I say. "That's got to be it!"

So, I start to think "where is the place I will never remember", and my answer is instinctive as I find myself staring at the pockets of an old coat that I never even wear. I check the pockets and in the left one find the keys. Winning!

"Catch me now, Cardinal", I chant, "catch me now!".
"You'll never work out what happens next", the Cardinal replies, but I know I will.
"The Devil himself! It has to be…".

I rush to the front door and scream "No, no" just as there is an almighty crash outside the front door that I am convinced the whole world must be able to hear. The Devil is trying to kick my door down, and no mistake, but I stand my ground, forcing the door back on him. The door survives and so do I, hinges and locks intact, simply because I got there fractionally first to repel the attack before it started. Henry is barking furiously behind me, and I realise how brave a hound can be. I am not alone, and this is a fight to the last!

It's obvious by now just how arrogant the Cardinal is, because the Devil was obviously supposed to kick the door down in a very physical way, and I have no idea what would have happened to me if he had succeeded. And I certainly don't want to find out! So the Cardinal's plan hasn't worked, but still he comes after me, taunting me about having no chance of survival, whilst he swings his spiked ball and chain, informing me of how many tortured souls he has killed with it. His favourite pastime is visiting the bowels of Hell expressly for this purpose apparently, and that is where I am going too.

Angels, Cleopatra and Psychosis

"Well, then, I'm living there already aren't I?", I say, and our confrontation continues.

Rock'n'roll is mesmeric in many ways and *Achtung Baby* is no exception. I realise that the Cardinal is swinging his ball and chain to its rhythms, and of course I know the music far better than he does. Or at least I think I do.

"Oh no you don't", he says. "I know everything you ever listen to, young man, so I most certainly know this".
"But you're not very good at dancing are you?", I taunt back.

I realise by now that I am starting to have the time of my life, for this is a confrontation I will never forget, and I am dancing as I have never danced before as the spiked ball and chain is aimed at my arms, my legs, and of course my head. Metaphysical or not, it whistles every time it goes past.

And then I really am frightened. Just at the end of *The Fly*, I dance myself to a full stop petrified as the Cardinal brings his ball and chain torture routine to an end.

I am standing directly in front of four Horsemen of the Apocalypse, each one rearing up at me as their riders try and scythe into me with their swords. As *Achtung Baby* continues into *She Moves In Mysterious Ways*, I am beginning to wonder whether playing it was such a good idea, but then what is done is done. More to the point, what to do now? The Cardinal was laughing loudly.

"Do you still feel being sworn to save Romancia is a good idea, Michael?", he says, and in the way he intones "Michael" I realise immediately how much he really does vehemently hate me.

"But why me?", I ask. "This isn't fair!".

"Of course it isn't fair Michael, because I don't want it to be. And neither does God Michael, and if you think Leonardo and Michelangelo have worked out our true plans then you are definitely mistaken. Our true plan is to crucify you and make the world go dark Michael. That way the world shall live in ignorance again, and we shall regain our powers".

This sounded truly terrifying, but I have four Horsemen to worry about, until I quickly realise they are effectively controlled by the Cardinal's thoughts.

"You will be dragged through the streets after the lights go out on the planet Michael, and people will not of course understand it is not you who are to blame"

"But what have I done to deserve this?", I asked.

"You will have made mistakes you cannot yet contemplate Michael, and in allying yourself to Leonardo and Michelangelo you have already made your first two. You will be forced to climb the Cross yourself Michael, and nailed to it in no uncertain terms. And this time the whole operation will be filmed Michael, so everyone on the planet will see it happen. My powers will be absolute!".

Angels, Cleopatra and Psychosis

A supernatural horse's hoof at this point seemed to break free from the control of its evil rider and I was struck a fearful blow to the left of my jaw bone. I fell to the ground but immediately got up again, only for what I can only describe as an astonishing surge of electricity to rise through my body from the floor, like the eruption of a volcano. It felt as if my head was about to explode, but I managed to put my hands on the top of my skull before the surge of electricity got there itself – I could see it all quite clearly through the reflection in the lounge window – and perhaps that is what saved me. All I remember is shouting "No, no" again, as I stood watching myself glow bright red. It looked like I had turned into the Devil himself.

Everything went quiet. The four Horsemen had vanished, and there was no sign of the Cardinal, although I knew he must still be around somewhere. What on earth had just happened? After perhaps five minutes I had stopped glowing red and my body seemed to return to normal. Not even my clothes were singed but I had no doubt that I had effectively been on fire. I looked at Henry, who had cowered in his basket the moment the four Horsemen had arrived, and he now walked slowly towards me with his tail between his legs, walking all around me. He was obviously frightened and concerned about me, but equally to the point I realised he hadn't been for a walk all day, and then I looked at the clock on the wall.

It was 3am.

And Henry was right. I got the feeling that he was telling me that going out into York on such a night was at least as safe as staying in the house, and after the experiences I'd been through, I entirely agreed. So that's what I did. I took Henry for a walk around York at 3am.

"You can't go out Michael", said the Cardinal as I put on Henry's lead. "That will be death".
"Then I'll die then" I replied.

The Cardinal this time was a whisper in my ear, not even a presence I could sense in the room, and I realised that he was obviously capable of spying on me any time he liked. How much about me did he know I wondered?, but then what was there to know? What had I ever really done wrong for instance?, and if he knew all my likes and dislikes for example, then I figured I knew them better than he did. I thought about the past actions of my life constantly, and maybe the Cardinal heard it all, but on the other hand Michelangelo seemed to think it didn't matter, and I still trusted him. Nevertheless, as Henry and I walked to the front door, I did wonder if we would make it. Was the Cardinal strong enough to actually stop me going out of the house, and did he want to? Henry though seemed confident and was straining at the leash, although not as much as usual. We were hardly in for a sunny stroll by the river this time, were we?

I opened the front door to find there was no doubt it had been physically attacked. The brass handle on the outside had been broken off, which was going to make the door difficult to open again, so I decided to leave it only so far closed, and luckily it stuck in the door frame. The Devil's footprints had made indents into the wood, and I speculated that his feet must be long and skinny. Strangely, I could only see four toe prints, but then what did I know about Devils, and why did I assume he had five? But it was a relief to be outside, even if I didn't know what was going to happen next, and even if I knew that the Devil must be around somewhere waiting for me. Henry was reassuring though, and he looked up at me expectantly with his ears cocked. He was obviously paying full attention, which was fortunate, because I was feeling exhausted and simply lucky to be alive. Henry's eyes were translucent in the moonlight.

Was the Devil an electrical energy force?, I wondered, because I had no doubt that it was the Devil's energy that had attacked me through the floor and made me glow red. But Henry wanted his walk, and I decided not to speculate about the Devil simply because I didn't know enough. I would report back to Leonardo and we would figure the rest out from there. And I also decided not to look backwards as Henry and I walked along a row of terraced houses opposite the railway line because I very quickly realised that I had the Devil on my tail. I could hear his breathing, I could almost hear his footprints. I half wanted to know if he really was red, or whether he glowed in the dark, but there was no way I was going to be so stupid as to look backwards and find out. Henry and I would stay on our walk until the morning came, because I simply assumed that come sunlight my nightmare would be over, at least for one day at least, and then I could talk to Leonardo and Michelangelo again.

Michael Black

I was temporarily exhausted, and Henry looked after me those first early morning hours. We were attacked by a long haired white cat who sprang out of some rubbish bins with its hair standing on end, but Henry saw it off, and we made our way over the railway footbridge, past the back of Bootham Park mental hospital and were soon at the bottom of Monkgate. I have forgotten most of the road names in York we travelled that night, but I can remember the route remarkably well and could probably retrace it even now, thirteen years later. It sounds perverse, but I avoided well lit streets, and stuck to the darker ones. I was determined to challenge darkness, I had no other choice, and I wasn't going to let the Devil see I was frightened. And as our walk progressed, I got the distinct sound impression that He was limping, perhaps from his failed exertions trying to kick my door down! Hard luck on the Devil, and I started to realise that that must have been a significant victory for me, and what's more, it had all been down to timing. How on earth had I worked out that the Devil would be at my door there and then? But I had and I had survived.

As we walked York that night I was looking for a wall I could sit down against in some safety to think. The night was cool and dry, and I had cigarettes with me too, but for some reason with the Devil on my tail I didn't want to light one when I was still moving. And then a police car arrived with sirens blazing, and I got verbally frisked. What was I doing out at this hour? "Well, walking the dog of course!". Did I know there had been several burglaries that night? *No, I did not!* Was I sure? *Yes, I was positive. And did it look like I was carrying around stolen CD players, officer?* Henry

Angels, Cleopatra and Psychosis

started barking at the police officer at this point, for which I apologised, but I could understand his impatience. I'm sure he was looking for a wall to sit down against just as much as I was, and the police intervention was just totally un-needed.

Eventually a wall was found, a railway bridge wall with a good view down the main road it traversed in either direction. I sat down and started thinking about what had happened to me. Maybe Henry was doing much the same thing, but I doubt it. He just sat throughout with his ears in antennae mode and I have never seen a dog seem so *en garde* in my life. This time I had no questions to ask myself about whether I had been through a series of delusions or not. What had happened had been real and true and the blow to my jaw had hurt. I had definitely met the invisible Cardinal again, and seen four Horsemen of the Apocalypse, but beyond that what did it all mean? After all, I wasn't even sure how many Horsemen of the Apocalypse there are prophesied in the Bible. But I did know I had been informed my fate was public crucifixion for future mistakes I couldn't possibly yet contemplate, and I also knew the Cardinal wanted the world to go dark again. Well, I wasn't settling for crucifixion, and I certainly wasn't settling for a world gone dark again, not least because it seemed to me that it was quite dark enough already. So I was in a state of warfare with the Cardinal, but then I knew that already, and I also knew my bonds to Leonardo and Michelangelo remained unbroken. And of course Romancia must be freed at all costs, so I felt like a man temporarily alone with a loyal hound beside him, that's all. Well, I thought, there are worse fates than that. And by now it must have been at least one hour from when Henry and I had left the house, so that was one less more hour of darkness that night to live through.

And I determined that if the threat was crucifixion I was going to raise the stakes all the way. "My God, why haste thou forsaken me". I remembered my conversations with Leonardo about that despairing line of Christ's, and found myself thinking about my own father, stroke ridden and crippled in a wheel chair. He didn't look dissimilar to the Victorian God on a cloud for that matter! Bald as well! My father's manic rages had to be seen and heard to be believed, and I came to realise how similar they were to those of the cruel and angry God of the Old Testament. And surely, having a God (my own father) crippled in a wheel chair with a stroke and a plastic valve in his heart was just one step beyond the God Leonardo insisted was actually Charles Darwin Himself stuck at ground level? Was my own father God, I found myself wondering? *I know it sounds mad, but it was making sense to me at the time*. If so, his son had a serious argument with him! I was not being crucified by anyone, or in anyone's cause. That night the love of both my mother and father as normal parents seemed to be impossible to imagine, and I found it impossible also to imagine that I had ever been the product of any impassioned or erotic, or caring, loving lovemaking. For some reason I felt like the child of rape, and felt stone cold inside as a consequence. My heart shrank.

And then God starting talking to me, and it wasn't a pleasant experience. "You are my Son alright", He said, "and you will die a hideous death". "Who are you? And why?" I countered, getting up immediately. "You are old and past it and knackered, Whoever you are, and I'm going to win. You won't crucify me!". "Try and stop me", said God. "Are you my father?", I asked, and "of course I am!" came the answer, as I realised the question had been pointless asking. "I am everyone's Father, my Son".

Having your imagination attacked by God is impossible to exactly describe, and I am not going to try. But the worst thing about it isn't that you can't get rid of the thunderous voice inside your own head. The worst thing is that your whole brain seems to expand inside your skull until a point is reached when you think your head will explode. I let go of Henry's lead and held my head as if to resist the expansion inside. "I am not Jesus Christ", I shouted, "I will not be crucified". "I know you are not Jesus, but you still will be" said God, laughing cruelly, "your name is Michael, and this time it will be even worse".

I went on the attack. I had no choice, it seemed like do or die.

"I am not being crucified!", I screamed. "I believe in Romancia, and I am working with Leonardo and Michelangelo to steal all power from you. I am going to kill you!".
"Kill me!", said God, "that's not possible". He laughed again.
"I am the Rebel!", I screamed, "the bringer of love and justice".

I thought of thinking of my own conception again. And I realised my mother's name was Mary!

"And I don't like the Virgin Mary either!", I screamed. "Frigid bitch!".

And I thought of all the world's starving and war torn children, in all the God forsaken shanty towns all over the planet's surface. I have never been so angry in my life.

"I am the child of rape and slaughter", I screamed, "and we will win! Romancia will be the wind of love and a new world will be born".

And then I felt wrapped in warmth by war torn and starving children the world over. They were knee high spirits to me, standing by me in adversity and they meant it. I felt the power of love.

And then I met the police again. Except this time it was a relief in a way. And for whatever reason, God had decided to leave my imagination to myself and was no longer tyrannising me. The policeman was a beat-bobby, and was clearly simply concerned.

"Are you alright?", he said.
"Yes, yes, I'm fine", I replied.
"You don't seem it, to be honest you know. Not the way you were screaming! You can't wake everyone up like that".
"There's no houses around here".

Angels, Cleopatra and Psychosis

If I was going to end up in Bootham Park mental hospital, it was not going to be tonight. I just wanted to go home and get some sleep. So I said so.

"What's your name and address?".
"Michael Black". I gave my address and then added "this is my dog Henry. I couldn't sleep, we've been for a walk, and now I'm going home".

The policeman wrote it all down and let me go.

"Take care", he said. And he stroked Henry gently.

I started walking again, and saw a neon sign at a petrol station saying "OPEN 24 HOURS" gleaming in the distance. And then I realised it was getting lighter. Somehow I had survived, and I was confident I was going to survive the walk home. And Henry no longer seemed the least bit concerned about anything. Added to which, I didn't feel the Devil was on my tail any more. In fact, I had forgotten at precisely what point I'd forgotten to worry about Him. Probably during my argument with God I suppose.

And then I realised I had forgotten about the invisible Cardinal too, but only when he started whispering in my ear.

"You'll be the last person left alive on earth Michael. And that's if you win. You'll have no one to talk to and no one to breed with…".
"Nonsense. I don't believe you. Leave me alone".
"There's not much chance of that".

"Tell me something new. I'm not bothered, and I want some sleep".

By the time I reached my front door again it must have been about 5am and the dawn was more than on its way. It was the most glorious dawn I had ever seen, after by far the longest night I had ever lived through. I was totally exhausted, and Henry made straight for his basket as well.

I walked upstairs and into the office-bedroom.

"Still alive then", said Leonardo. "Well done".
"Not that we had any doubts", said Michelangelo.
"You won't believe what I've been through", I said, exhausted.
"It doesn't matter for now. Just get some sleep", said Leonardo.

So I did. But I was too invigorated to really sleep and woke up at around 8-30am.

I switched on the PC, only to find it had completed crashed and all the files on it were corrupted. *Was it the work of the Cardinal I wondered?* But it didn't matter. It would cause me hassle rebuilding the machine, but all the stage play and novel files I valued were double saved on floppy disks anyway. I didn't care.

And then I pulled open the curtains, expecting a brand new day, only to find that little red devils were staring through the window at me and trying to threaten me in open daylight! After the night I had just been through it seemed hilarious, I just laughed, and I also had to tell someone, so I immediately rang up my old school friend Richard, then working in the Agriculture department of Edinburgh University.

But Richard obviously didn't see the funny side, and was clearly concerned about my state of mental health. He told me he was immediately getting in the car to come and see me and would be with me in about four hours. He was as good as his word. When Richard arrived, he immediately rang my mother.

It was obvious that Bootham Park mental hospital wasn't very far away on the horizon.

Interlude

Well, well, well now! You've now read two chapters concerning my supposed collapse of mental health during 1993 and 1994. I say *supposed* because there are other ways of looking at these things. Yes, it is true as established in the *Intro* that my life was going badly and I was under a lot of stress because of that – unemployment, a failing marriage and the pain of losing daily contact with my young son Robert when the marriage finally went in 1994 don't help anyone's state of mental health. But it's also true that they don't necessarily mean you're hypomanic either, as I was initially diagnosed by psychiatrists in a mental hospital in Mansfield, Nottinghamshire, after meeting Michelangelo for the first time for instance.

That's my opinion anyway. Psychiatrists see the world through the eyes of biologically driven medical psychiatric theory and also see the re-establishment of sanity as largely dependent on the administration of various psychiatric drugs, be they mood stabilisers such as Lithium Carbonate or Sodium Valproate (in its two preparations Epilim and Depacote), or the umpteen anti-psychotics in tablet and depot injection form now on the market. The fact that the patient (and most patients disagree with their diagnosis in my experience) might well see their situation in different terms is not something I've ever found a psychiatrist to be interested in hearing about. The patient is presumed not to know what they are talking about, and if the patient disagrees with the psychiatrist, then all that happens is the patient gets notes written about them saying they have "no insight" into their condition. The patient is not the doctor, and the doctor knows best.

Except of course in 1993 and 1994, starting in Mansfield, and on various psychiatric wards thereafter (the Victorian Parkside asylum, Macclesfield and another modern unit in Harlow, Essex now immediately spring to mind) I was the doctor, although a doctor of a different kind to the psychiatrists. I was a doctor of philosophy from the elite University of Cambridge, as I have already explained. Now I was and remain to this day incredibly proud of this fact, and as it quickly became apparent to me how complacent and lazy most psychiatrists are, I started to question their judgements about me in bolder and bolder ways, not least because all most psychiatrists seem to do for a living is almost randomly choose the drugs they put you on from a cursory glance through BNF (British National Formulary), having used the DSM (Diagnostic Statistical Manual, now on version 5) to work out what illness they thought you have or had in the first place.

And I was a piss taking disruptive psychiatric patient as well, thinking of myself as the Jack Nicholson character thinks of himself in *One Flew Over the Cuckoo's Nest*. Nicholson was my daily inspiration for my next piece of ironic performance art on the wards of Bootham Park and Westerdale Ward in York as I now remember them, and as I also now remember the "half-way house" of Red Roofs in York they put me in after that as well. But whilst I had the odd good laugh and fought back every time they told me I was mad, I was also mad enough to tell the psychiatrists I spoke to (and I remember one particularly unpleasant female bully called Dr. Susan P. Shaw in York) about my experiences of meeting Michelangelo, Leonardo da Vinci and the invisible Cardinal, as well as also telling them about the strange dreams I was starting to have at the time about trying to kill the Greek god Zeus. I wanted to debate with the psychiatrist whether Zeus was the same or a different *personae* from our own Christian God, but psychiatrists never debate philosophical questions like that. That's the kind of thing doctors of philosophy do! The psychiatrists just thought I was long gone and going further...

The result was that the original diagnosis of hypomania, which I had objected to, was changed to one of schizophrenia, which I objected to even more, but that's life! And the drugs were changed too. I can't remember the drugs they used for the hypomania, but they weren't too debilitating, save for the first administration of Haloperidol in Mansfield, which was temporary if memory serves me correctly. The drugs they used on me for schizophrenia, however, were both horrendous. First Largactil, and then, when I continued to argue the case for my essential sanity and insist on the genuine and non-psychotic nature of the experiences described in *A Meeting With Michelangelo* and *Devil At The Door*, a depot injection drug called Clopixol, which made me increasingly comatose, walk around like a zombie, and also, and very depressingly, made me impotent (I have also been on Risperdal Consta injections by the way, and that makes me comatose and impotent as well, despite the fact that it claims to be a modern "atypical" side-effect free drug).

Angels, Cleopatra and Psychosis

My life was going nowhere and I was in a mess. I hadn't yet realised that if you're having so-called psychotic experiences or hearing voices for example (as many psychiatric patients do), then if you want to get out of the mental hospital fast (which I did), it is best practice simply not to open up to the nurses and psychiatrists about the experiences you are going through at all. They're not interested in exceptional experience, never record it properly, and besides, I've come to the conclusion it's mainly your own business, unless, as a writer like me, you choose to make your experiences intentionally public thereafter.

But 1994 and 1995 were both years of psychiatric confinement, first on Section 2s (for 28 days), and then, after the change of diagnosis to schizophrenia, on Section 3s (which are for up to six months, and for me always meant six months, and were also then renewed). I was on the locked ward of Westerdale in York, and then, nine months later after several very boring months at the Red Roofs "halfway house", I was finally released, so long as I went to live with my mother in my home town of Wilmslow, Cheshire, where I had once attended Gorsey Bank Primary School and then Wilmslow Grammar School before going on to York University in 1980 to do my first degree.

But I was still on Clopixol injections, administered by my Community Psychiatric Nurse Nigel Bailey, based at the Parkside asylum in Macclesfield, I was still comatose and still impotent. I felt I had no valid life at all. I was the zombie himself.

Michael Black

It was my mother who started to complain to the authorities about the use of Clopixol, arguing that surely there must be other less debilitating drugs that could be used. The authorities at first argued that one of the reasons for the depot injection was that they didn't trust me to take drugs in tablet form on a regular basis, given my opposition to their diagnosis of my condition, but eventually they relented and agreed to put me on the tablet form drug Clozaril in October 1995, provided I agreed to return to the Parkside asylum, Macclesfield, for one month whilst the switchover of drugs was made.

Clozaril, next to Clopixol, was a dream to be on. I almost immediately stopped being comatose, my normal co-ordination returned and so did my sexual potency. After two years of psychiatric hell I decided to just take the drug every day, forget about arguments with psychiatry and the diagnosis of schizophrenia which I still found so offensive, and just concentrate on rebuilding my life.

I got a job working in a Wilmslow petrol station in the April of 1996, and was to have no real contact again with psychiatry until the summer of 2001, save seeing my CPN Nigel Bailey once a month. I spent two and a half years working at the petrol station, also retraining as a librarian at Manchester Metropolitan University during this time. Then I got an 18 month job working for Waterstone's bookshop at Manchester airport, and I also moved out of my mother's house to live in my own at first rented house in Macclesfield in August 1998. Finally, I got a job as an assistant librarian at Macclesfield College in late 1999, but I

Angels, Cleopatra and Psychosis

never really thought librarianship was for me. By this time, ever the various mind, I'd also retrained as a website designer at Manchester City College, and was employed as a website designer by Stockport Metropolitan Borough Council Education Authority in the year 2000, where I was to remain for the next five years.

There was no new woman in my life, but, other than that, I was rebuilding my life to good effect, so much so that Dr. Chung, my GP, refused to renew my DLA (Disability Living Allowance) in 1998, and also wrote to my psychiatrist questioning the diagnosis of schizophrenia in the first place. But I only found that out years later when, having paid for the privilege, I assembled all my own psychiatric notes (those written by nurses and psychiatrists), and got Jayne Phillips of the charity Macclesfield Mind to read them for me whilst I was preparing the material for this book.

In 1998, I also started writing again, after my play about Beethoven, originally commissioned by the Arts Council in late 1991, and now called *Panharmonicon*, was re-commissioned by the West End producer Peter Wilson. And I completed my experimental novel about the relationship between Beethoven and Napoleon *Crossing Out The Emperor*, which I had originally started working on alone in York in 1993. My play *The Amber Room*, written in 1992, was produced on the London fringe in the Spring of 1998, and I also finally completed two other plays, *Madame Viardot* and *The Wedding*, both of which had been on my mind since before my initial mental breakdown in 1993. All this work and more then found its way onto the website I designed to display it, www.mwblack.co.uk, where it remains to this day, and I also did other freelance website work during this period, designing the Macclesfield Voluntary Organisations website for instance, paid for and proposed by the European Union themselves, the EU being an organisation I remain proud of working for to this day. They were good employers and they paid well as well!

By the late 1990s, my life had a new presumed stability about it, and new friendships were being made, with the likes of my near Wilmslow contemporary Nick Stubbs (also my partner in website design), and also with my boss at Stockport MBC, Mike Partridge, although this friendship, which lasts to this day, would take longer to develop.

And then in the summer of 2001, my father's partner Peggy (my mother and father separated when I was 11 years old in 1974) tried to kill herself with an overdose of morphine. Now not only do I have no sympathy with suicide cases (for my position read that of Albert Camus in *The Myth of Sisyphus*), but this act of desperation plunged the family into a wider extended crisis that was to last several years. My father was a stroke ridden cripple of 74 with a plastic heart valve and a pacemaker to boot and incapable of looking after himself. He had lived in a wheelchair since 1982, and needed the provision of expensive private nursing homes, as it soon became clear did Peggy herself, although for that it was not my family paying the bill. But without Peggy around, it was soon my mother who was looking after all my father's affairs again, a necessity perhaps under the circumstances, but nevertheless a fact that deeply irritated me. What was a woman who had left a man in 1974 doing still looking after him twenty seven years later? The answer is simply, as I also knew, that there was no one else to do the job, and my mother must have felt her life greatly compromised. My father, already an alcoholic, complained of the standards of the first nursing home Mum found for him in Mobberley, Cheshire, not least because the staff restricted his drinking bouts, and he became, quite simply, a constant problem, something he had always been anyway, but this time on an escalating scale. Every time I took him out for a lunch time drink at the weekends I would look at him wishing he would just fuck off and die. My mother started to talk about him more and more, which irritated me more and more, and I came to hate the guts of the very NHS that had given him the plastic heart valve and pacemaker at *immense* cost in the first place. Without those he would have been dead years ago I remember thinking! My mother is very healthy, but she is also only one year younger than my father, and I also became terrified that she might die first, leaving me with the creatively debilitating responsibilities of trying to look after my father, something I was aware I would resent even more, because in my opinion he was already living an essentially whisky fuelled pointless and self-indulgent life anyway.

Then my father had a fall and broke his hip and caught the killer bug MRSA in hospital. I prayed it would kill him, but it didn't. The NHS saw to that, and patched his hip back up again as well, and I came to hate the NHS even more for doing so. And the terror of my mother dying first remained. I knew I could never be happy until my father was dead. And the sooner the better.

Eternity On Bollin Ward

As I have said in the Interlude, between 1995 and 2001 I got my life back together again, and had minimal contact with Macclesfield mental health services. So unbeknown to me were the great changes within Macclesfield mental health during this time. But the old Victorian asylum of Parkside was closed down, and a new purpose built unit of four new wards was built called the Millbrook Unit, close to the General Hospital itself. This opened in 1997. The extensive grounds of the old Parkside asylum are now an upwardly mobile housing estate, something many people within mental health resent. The physical space once available to the patients has been taken away. Nevertheless, in some ways the Millbrook Unit represents a serious advance over the facilities that were available at Parkside. At Parkside you slept in horrible communal dormitories with creaking iron bedsteads and straw mattresses, whereas all the wards at the Millbrook Unit provide patients with their own individual bedroom, all of which came as a very pleasant shock to me when I first found out about it! The privacy of your own room always means you can escape the psychotics around you when it all gets too much and yet another TV gets smashed to pieces.

The Millbrook Unit consists of four wards, A, B, C and D, if you like. Adelphi Ward is an acute ward built around a central open to the elements courtyard, which can be a very pleasant place to relax during the summer, and there is another acute ward, Bollin Ward, directly above Adelphi Ward, which conforms to exactly the same architectural plan, except that since it is upstairs, there is nowhere for the patients to go outside. I have known people live an entirely indoor life on Bollin Ward for as long as six months. Hell. Then there is Croft Ward, the ward for the elderly, and finally there is Dane Ward, the ward for the long stay most serious cases.

Despite increased recent expenditure on the NHS, the acute Bollin Ward was closed down in November 2006, so now the only acute ward is Adelphi Ward.

My own first psychiatric admission to the Millbrook Unit was to Adelphi Ward in the summer of 2001, and I remember both Nick Stubbs and Mike Partridge coming to see me the first weekend I was there. I was still taking Clozaril, but for some reason went very high, in a way that conforms to the original diagnosis of hypomania far more than the subsequent diagnosis of schizophrenia. I was put on a Section 3, but was only on the ward for about a month before being released again, at which point I went on holiday to Paris for ten days. But that's another story. I came back high again, and was re-sectioned, but again only for about a month, and by the end of the summer of 2001 the whole episode had been dismissed as something of a blip, so I went back to my job as a website designer at Stockport MBC, and forgot all about it.

Perhaps I should have paid more attention, because the Millbrook Unit was to become a regular feature of my life over the next five years. I have been on Adelphi Ward more times than I now care to

Angels, Cleopatra and Psychosis

remember for example, although this statement must be qualified by the fact that by about 2003 I was so unhappy in my job that I decided I would rather take sick leave and live on a psychiatric ward and write than actually go to work! I have at least seven notebooks written under such circumstances, developing a lot of the material for Stealing Heaven From God, and also containing the first attempts of a stage play I started to write first in 2000, about the mental breakdown of Picasso's mistress Dora Maar, when he left her in 1943. But it is only this year in 2007 that I have finally finished the play, entitled The Minotaur, and I put a great deal of my mental health problems 2001-2006, the date of my last admission, down pure and simply to writers' block. But try telling that to a psychiatrist...

But this chapter is set on Bollin Ward in 2003, the first time I had been admitted there. It tells the story of the reasons behind it all, and what happened next, but one more thing must be added for the context. By this time (and it is a very long story), Leonardo da Vinci, Michelangelo and myself had all decided that my own father, John Black, was in fact God the Father Himself in disguise...

I was at home in the computer room, on the first floor of my house, working on notes for my Dora Maar play. Suddenly there was a loud crack of thunder, and a voice boomed from above Heaven itself.

"I am Cleopatra, Michael. How dare you write in your book that I live in Paradise. And you've also written down that you've had dream sex with me when you haven't. You will pay for this!".

I knew I was in trouble immediately, but also somewhere delighted. Cleopatra was a woman, a myth and a legend of immense stature after all, and one that had fascinated me ever since I had read her book on Egyptian cosmetics when I was an eight year old boy.

"So you do live in Paradise?", I asked.

"Yes, above Heaven, in a dimension you don't understand. Stop thinking about Dora Maar Michael and learn your fate. You are far, far too young to understand anything about this, and I don't care about your God either. I have different battles in mind. Stop thinking about Dora Maar!".

So I stopped writing, not to obey Cleopatra, but because it was obvious I had to pay attention. I went downstairs to the living room, found my cigarettes and lit one. What was going to happen next? And I was itching to find out! I had written in *Stealing Heaven From God* that Cleopatra reigns in Paradise, and the next thing you know, she's talking to me! On the other hand, she was clearly very angry, and saying I'd had dream sex with a woman of that kind of power had obviously been a big mistake. *Or had it?* I remembered writing the very words myself, but had it been as a kind of challenge to her? Cleopatra had always been a fantasy of mine after all. If I hadn't written I'd had dream sex in Paradise with Cleopatra, would she have declared herself at all?

Cleopatra appeared in the lounge before me. She wore the robes of an ancient Queen, her headdress regal but understated. It was dusk and getting dark. There was an immediate sense of *frisson* between us.

"I've been watching you Michael" said Cleopatra, "and you are even more stupid than Michelangelo and Leonardo. So you think your father is God do you? Well, I don't care either way, but I think you'll find you haven't won all your battles with Him yet. If you had, He'd be dead".
"Now listen here", said Michelangelo, sitting on my sofa, "you can't treat Michael like this. He hasn't published his book yet, and he has a perfect right to write what he wants on his own word processor in the freedom of his own home!".

Of course, according to liberal sensibilities, Michelangelo was entirely right about this, but it was obvious Cleopatra didn't see things that way, and anyway, I reflected that as I had been making notes for the very book you are reading now, I had been aware of forces behind me watching every word that was written. I'd just ignored them I suppose and got on with it. As so often, I was now in more peril than previously, but how often had that been the case over the previous ten years? God, the invisible Cardinal and now Cleopatra constantly dismissed me as far too young and pilloried Leonardo and Michelangelo, but somehow we all seemed to survive until our next adventure. So far, I had no doubt we would do the same again. And then I started to change my mind.

"I am sending spaceships to destroy the earth!", screamed Cleopatra. "My battles are ones you can barely imagine Michael, and it suits my purposes to destroy it all".

I must admit I was terrified now. That was a serious threat!

"None of you understand anything Michael!", she continued. "You are just romantics out of your depth. You all keep up your argument with God, but have you yourself ever met God Michael? You think God is your Father but you have no idea of His true power! And I am far more powerful than He is anyway. I am the Sun Goddess!".

At this I was naturally speechless. Thunder cracked, and I looked out of the window. It was dark, pitched dark and raining. Damp Macclesfield in November writ large. I thought about spaceships destroying the earth, and then I did something very stupid. I switched on the television.

"Oh, you won't see it happen on a television set!", laughed Cleopatra. "And people do get very frightened when I speak Michael, once every few hundred years. The earth will be destroyed, the sun will go out, and everyone will know it is your fault Michael. You are young, arrogant, and unbelievably stupid. You have no chance".

I still didn't believe this, but I did know I was in serious trouble. And then worse!

Angels, Cleopatra and Psychosis

"My imagination is much bigger than yours, son", thundered a voice. It could only be one person. God Himself, and it was.
"Hello Dad", I said.
"Hello, son" came the reply.

And I was terrified now. The voice completely surrounded me, but it was inside my head as well. How on earth was I to escape my fate this time? I had managed to survive spiritual attack many times, but this time I really was up against it, and Michelangelo was nowhere to be seen or heard. He doubtless had his own battles to fight, as I had mine.

"I only live in a crippled old body sitting in a wheelchair when it suits me, Michael", said God, "and now I am free. You should have physically murdered me whilst you could, but the plastic heart valve has kept me alive beyond the Last Judgement, and now I am free! I was going to re-make the world anew, and now the Sun Goddess will destroy it as she has always wanted to".

I decided to fight back.
"Dad, I said, you're in Barclay Park Nursing Home, Mobberley, Cheshire, England, and you're pissed and drunk on whisky again. Get out of my head!".

"I'm not pissed", said God, "I'm legless again, that's all. But then I've been legless effectively ever since my stroke in 1982. You can't explain these things to people Michael, but I am going to make sure everyone knows the destruction of the universe is your fault. The sun will go out Michael. The earth will be destroyed by spaceships and live in darkness. And I am going to make you walk the world in penance. Get out of this house!".

I had no intention of doing any such thing, and was still searching for a way out. I obviously didn't have one, but my survival instinct took over. So I went back up the stairs to the kitchen, made a cup of tea, and then made a decision to try and sleep through the night. Did I really believe the sun would go out? Did I really believe Cleopatra was sending space ships to destroy the world or believe that she was the Sun Goddess? I needed time to think about it all, and I needed evidence as well. Evidence of the sun shining again, and as I looked out of the window, it did seem a long shot, but then this was south Manchester in the winter at night, hardly the sunniest of climes.

I was more worried about the voice of God. "My imagination is bigger than yours, son" he had said to me before, and it certainly seemed that way. On the other hand, if I was trapped inside his force field – and that is how it felt – then it was bound to seem that way, and the question became how to get outside it? This was a battle if ever there was one, and I still wasn't giving in.

I climbed the stairs to the second floor bedroom, but it only got worse. The invisible Cardinal was waiting for me, more powerful than I had ever seen him, and it was obvious there was no way I was going to bed. I was beginning to feel dead in the water, and

Angels, Cleopatra and Psychosis

was by now trembling with fear. I looked at the clock. It said 8-30pm.

"You are going to walk out of this house, Michael", said the Cardinal, "and walk the world. There is no way back for you, and everyone will know it is you who has challenged the Sun Goddess and destroyed the planet. You will be stoned, and lashed, buggered by rapists, nailed and crucified in the end, and you cannot escape me now. So take off your clothes".

The rain lashed against the window. And I did as I was told, standing naked on my bedroom carpet.

"Look at you. You wouldn't live long anyway. You have destroyed your own promise with this ridiculous fight of yours against us Michael. Where is Leonardo now Michael? Where is Michelangelo? Will Romancia ever escape from Hell? Of course not! You are dead and nailed Michael. And you smoke too much, and a once fine figure has run to fat. And you are flat footed and slow. As for me I will survive. The world may go dark, but Rome will rule that darkness, and I shall be Pope at last. We will let everyone know when you are crucified Michael. This is the fate that awaits anyone who disobeys us...".

Now, me and the Cardinal go back a long way as you know, and although I felt desperate, and could see I was going to have to try and walk the world (an impossibility from Macclesfield anyway, Great Britain being an island), one thing did strike me about this speech, namely that I do not have flat feet, I have very well arched feet. So although I wasn't going to argue with the Cardinal there and then, I was thinking that if he was still exaggerating, then he must be overstating his case. So naked in my bedroom, I stood my ground. And, I was determined, if I was going to walk out in the rain and darkness, it was not going to be naked!

"I have heard my God speak at last", said the Cardinal, "and He is my only master! Get out of this house Michael, and face up to your dreadful fate!".

And then help arrived at last! I looked up to the high ceiling of the bedroom, and saw a beautiful female angel, wings outspread, hovering over me. Her auburn hair hung down partly covering her face, and then she landed on the floor and stood immediately behind me.

"Don't do anything the Cardinal says Michael. Stand your ground", she said.

And then she put her arms around my waist.
"Hello Michael", she said. "I'm the angel Jana come to save you".
And then she gently kissed the nape of my neck.

"Get out of here!", said the Cardinal.
"Try me", replied my rescuer of the night. "I can stand my ground too. Don't take me on Cardinal. I love this man". She held me closer. "Michael. There is a way out of this, but you must act fast and trust me. I have other plans. And you must look smart. So get showered and shaved and put your best suit on. Then we order a taxi to Manchester airport and get a flight to Paris whilst we still can. Believe me, we still have a chance".

Angels, Cleopatra and Psychosis

I didn't argue. I was already naked, so I grabbed a towel and was in the shower in no time, in love with Jana as I had never been in love with a normal woman in my life! An angel had rescued me! I couldn't believe it! But before I knew it, the Cardinal was in the shower with me, his hands gripped my genitals until he shrunk them to the size of a small boy's.

"This time, I am serious", said the Cardinal, "and you are not escaping Michael".

It was no use. The Cardinal had me this time. This time I now felt truly defeated, and my capacity to resist further just evaporated. I went back up to the bedroom still naked and wet from the shower, and looked full on at Jana, as she looked back at me. Her wings were spread, but I could see she was worried.

"I know darling", she said, "I know. Perhaps they've got you now".

And then she vanished. I felt cold, but some slight will to resist was still within me, so I thought of an act of defiance and put a jumper on and a pair of blue track suit bottoms, and that's all. And I just stood there.

"Take those clothes off", said the Cardinal.

But I kept them on. And then I walked down the stairs and out of the house, closing the front door behind me without any keys. I was also without money or credit cards or even a pair of glasses. And I was also barefoot.

It was cold and wet and windy and dark, and I walked down the Hurdsfield Road hill, expecting the doors of the terraced houses to be opened at any moment by their angry occupants as they started to stone me to death. But the streets were quiet, and there was even no noise coming out of the Flower Pot pub. Going down the hill towards Tescos, the rain increased, and I stopped, soaked, feeling like the loneliest man in the world. Jana had tried to save me, but the Cardinal had been too strong, and my fate was sealed.

"Don't stop", said the Cardinal, as I realised he was right behind me. "You must walk the world, and so far you've only walked a few hundred yards".

I started walking again, turning left on to the Silk Road, but then I stopped again, thinking "what is the point of this?". My life was over anyway, so what did I care for the Cardinal's commands now? My end was obviously going to be bloody and messy whatever I did, so I might as well disobey him one more time. I was still on the point of utter desperation, but then God did something very stupid. Just as I was pondering the impossibility of fighting His imaginative power, His voice thundered at me,

"You must learn to love the Virgin Mary. It is your only hope. In that can still lie your salvation".

And I knew immediately I had to refuse, so I did.

Angels, Cleopatra and Psychosis

"Fuck off!" I screamed, and I meant it.

I was cold, wet, effectively homeless and penniless, but I started walking again at this point, thinking only that I was not going to allow the Cardinal to run a world of darkness whilst the ignorant prayed before the Madonna once again. And I decided to ignore everything the Cardinal said. I knew what I needed. Somehow I needed to find breathing space. It was obvious that that was what Jana had been trying to find too, and we'd failed, but I believed she must still be around somewhere, and I started to think about what my real options were. I needed somewhere safe and warm, I needed a bed. By now I had turned right under the railway bridge and was walking down Sunderland Street, past Gio's pizzas. And still I hadn't met a soul. It might be dark and thunderous, and it felt like the whole world was peering at me from behind its windows, but on the other hand, God and the Cardinal had threatened me with being stoned and buggered by rapists, but it showed no signs of happening so far. So I kept walking, for some reason determined only to make it to Lowe St., where I planned to stop and just wait and see what happened to me next. So that is exactly what I did. I just stood on Lowe St. soaked, cold and lonely and awaited my fate. At the same time, it was also occurring to me that I wasn't that far from Adelphi ward, and I started to wonder whether they would let me in. For the first time in my life I desperately needed the right of asylum, and I knew it. The question was becoming, how to go about getting in?

Michael Black

"Michael, if you are thinking a mental hospital will help you now, you are badly mistaken", said the Cardinal.

I just ignored him and stood my ground. I was reminded of my night on the streets of York back in 1994, and I was reminded of the children of rape and slaughter too. They had sworn allegiance to me as I to them, and I was not going to let them down. Somehow I was going to survive all this. I was desperate for a cigarette, but I'd left those in the house as well. I had nothing, and for now I wasn't moving. I just stood barefoot in the rain on Lowe St., waiting to find out what was going to happen next.

And then a police car drew up. Two officers got out of it, one female, the other male, and the female one approached me. I was relieved. At the very least it was obvious they were going to put me in the back of the police car, and I would be out of the cold and rain. The woman police officer asked me my name and address, but I just said nothing, and immediately decided I was going to go on saying nothing for as long as possible. What else was there to say? How could I explain my night thus far to anyone? I knew only that I had to survive somehow until the sun came up again, if it ever did, and it seemed like a personal challenge. Could I survive that long?, for time in such situations can do very strange things, and I felt extremely weak and cold and lonely. And at the most it can only have been about 10pm that evening, so even assuming that the sun came up the next morning – and I might have to have a battle with Cleopatra about it first – there was still a very long way to go.

Angels, Cleopatra and Psychosis

In the back of the police car I soon was, reflecting how much I appreciated the police, particularly the conduct of the female officer. I was aware the Cardinal was in the car sitting next me, but I didn't care. This was already a triumph of my will against his, and I had decided I wasn't going to do anything as ridiculous as trying to walk the world for anyone! In which direction for a start! And over what mountain ranges? I knew I was still in deep trouble, but I didn't care. The back of a police car was better than Lowe St. in the rain.

I was wondering if I was heading for the police cells, but the police drove straight to A&E at Macclesfield District General Hospital, where they handed me over to a nurse. I was asked my name and address again, but I still refused to say anything, and was soon in a room on my own for what must have been 40 minutes at least. But it was warm, and I didn't care. The Cardinal was in there with me of course, but by now it was all becoming absurd between him and me, and I began to get the feeling that I was playing him one last time. He repeated his threats about stoning and buggery, and nailing and crucifixion, and then he started threatening me as he had in York in 1994, standing in front of me swinging his ball and chain, but I just sat in my chair and watched it all. At one point I even closed my eyes and tried to get some sleep, but decided that was too risky. I was profoundly knackered, but somehow I had to presently stay awake. Even if I said nothing, I had to stay aware and take nothing for granted.

Michael Black

Eventually a nurse came in and put a cup of tea down on a table. I just left it there and the nurse walked out again. And then a psychiatrist turned up, a woman who I'd never met before. She introduced herself as Dr. Galloway and asked me what I had been doing standing outside in the rain and so on, but I just said nothing. She must have asked me other questions, including name and address of course, but I replied to none of them, increasingly thinking "there is only one place I am going, and it's bound to be Adelphi ward, and I'll play it from there". And it was an interesting experience being anonymous, and somehow gave me an advantage. No one presently knew who I was, and I figured no one had so far put two and two together and worked out I was (to them) "Michael Black the schizophrenic". In some ways therefore I felt like a free man. I could have said anything, changed my name, whatever, but for now, the anonymity of silence suited me. And it was also the best way of conserving energy. Further, I knew from past experience that when you are profoundly knackered it is impossible to convince a psychiatrist you are basically OK, so there was no point trying. And anyway, I didn't want releasing, or driving back to my house to face God, the Cardinal and Cleopatra on my own again. I wanted the asylum of Adelphi ward more than anything, and I would take it from there.

Anyway, after another couple of hours waiting, Adelphi ward is effectively where I was taken, except the ward was full, so I was actually put on Bollin ward, another acute ward of exactly the same shape, plan and design, except for the fact that it is directly above Adelphi ward and therefore has no courtyard. But courtyards are for summer fun anyway, and I had no intention of going outside even if allowed, which I wouldn't have been. But I couldn't help wondering whether Leonardo and Michelangelo weren't still guarding the Adelphi courtyard as they had when I had been on it in 2001, and therefore Bollin ward too, as they said they always would be when it mattered, and it certainly mattered now. *What was I thinking?* I was thinking about Cleopatra and the sun going out and the end of the world and mass chaos and destruction, and I was also thinking that there was no way anyone was pinning all the blame on me. And I was also thinking about the seeming impossibility of defeating God by having an imagination bigger than His, I was thinking about his thunderous booming voice and how much I still hated Him! In fact for someone in a state so knackered, I was thinking far too much, and about far too many things!

I'd never been on Bollin ward before, but working out the place took five minutes since the layout was the same as Adelphi. There were no interesting games to play on this ward, I'd played them all before, and I was relieved when I was shown my room, luckily a single one. Not that I had any intention of sleeping in it for now, and I was soon to find out I wasn't going to be given the chance anyway, so after working out that the same TV station was playing in the smoking lounge, the non-smoking lounge and the so called tiny music room, I decided the best place to be was the smoking lounge and I just sat down in a chair. I was still refusing to speak, and I also decided to do without cigarettes, even if I could scrounge some, and also do without food and water too. I was going to see this out the hard way, my only challenge to the ultimate powers that be! Try me as a mere mortal, one far too young to understand these metaphysical power structures of time and space and the universe! *Try me and see what I can take!* My clothes were wet, but I was still alive, and I wasn't bothered for now about how long I was going to be on a psychiatric ward or whether I'd been sectioned or not. I'd met a female angel called Jana in Heaven's name, I did know that, and now I was feeling slightly safer, it did seem like another of those most extraordinary days!

In fact, if the world was effectively ending, and everyone thought it was my fault, then a psychiatric ward seemed a very good place to be! I could always plead insanity, after all!

The Cardinal of course was following me everywhere, but I was still ignoring him, including his constant reminders of having shrivelled and destroyed my manhood (which was most definitely true). And I was no longer actively fighting him. This was all about God and Cleopatra, and it all began to seem fascinating. Safe and warm, at least for now, all I wanted was a cigarette, but I was determined not to scrounge any, because I wanted to live on nothing for as long as possible, and see what I needed the most first. Further, I still believed in my allegiance to Leonardo and Michelangelo, and I knew they would be on the case somewhere. In fact, I worked out, they were probably at Barclay Park Nursing Home having it out in a straight confrontation with God my Father Himself! It was all beginning – though still terrifying – to seem like a very interesting situation to be in. I had discovered Cleopatra

Angels, Cleopatra and Psychosis

did live in Paradise after all, or so she said, and what's more, she was the Sun Goddess herself!. Well now, not even Leonardo had worked that one out!

I was mulling all the above over in my head, and quickly got bored of the smoking lounge, so I went for a walk around the corridors for about five minutes before coming back to the same place. The clocks read about 2am. And then the angel Jana suddenly appeared in the doorway, looking radiant and gorgeous with her free flowing auburn hair, even if she was only wearing jeans and a cream T-shirt with bare feet. She smiled at me, quickly spread her wings, put her left fore finger to her lips immediately, and then vanished again. I don't think even the Cardinal saw her – and I'm sure everyone one else on the ward most certainly didn't – but I most certainly did, so at last I started to feel reassured. I hadn't lost her after all, and Paris had not been our only chance!

That had been my one unspoken fear ever since I'd lost my manhood in the shower, and now I was beginning to be sure there was a way out of all of this. And I was fairly certain that Jana knew more about it than I did.

But I know more about Dr. Josef Goebbels than she does, my stage play *Pure Walking Evil* is all about him after all, and guess who turned up next? The man himself. Yes, that's right, I was soon in an audience with Dr. Josef Goebbels on Bollin ward of all places, and what's more, he had Adolph Hitler and Heinrich Himmler with him too. Well, it had always been obvious to me that the Cardinal was a Nazi of some description anyway, and now I had three more to deal with! What would they have to say for themselves now? And further, I was finding the chairs very uncomfortable by now, so I decided to sit on the floor and have my audience with them from there.

They were of course all spirits by the way, just as every other being of real importance in this book is a spirit, and just as before, they were invisible to the world, but I could see them as clear as day. I just didn't know where this was leading any more, but after seeing the angel Jana and knowing she was on the ward too, I just decided to relax. And I noticed immediately that Dr. Goebbels looked very badly burned (Dr. Goebbels' body was burnt with petrol after he shot himself in the Fuhrerbunker in 1945, but there wasn't enough petrol to finish the job). I decided it was best not to comment on this, and besides, I had no intention of breaking my silence for now, but suffice to say that Dr. Goebbels was not looking his best.

He stared at me, I stared back. I still said nothing, and it seemed to unnerve him, so the tactic seemed to be working and I kept on doing it. I wasn't dead yet.

Dr. Goebbels performed the Nazi salute.
"Heil Hitler!" he shouted.
"Heil Hitler!", I intoned back. I was taking the piss.

"Michael", said Dr. Goebbels. "None of this is good enough. Walking the world would have been preferable to this you know. You're a coward".

Angels, Cleopatra and Psychosis

I wasn't going to rise to this and still said nothing. I was more interested in self preservation! I decided just to listen sitting on the floor, and find out how much worse my fate was going to be now. Dr. Goebbels continued.

"I am a very senior devil Michael, senior in some respects to the Devil Himself, but I won't explain myself further. The world is to be plunged into darkness, a permanent blitzkrieg, so do you think I am unhappy about this? I like bloodshed Michael, I like tyranny and chaos, and the Cardinal shall be Pope at last, his ultimate ambition. But then who cares about that? How many tanks has the Pope got? Nevertheless I am pleased for the Cardinal, but I am not pleased with you. You cannot stay here Michael, I won't allow it. You've never been on Bollin Ward before and this is my kingdom. And if you try to stay here, I shall tell you what will happen. You will be given electric shock treatment to erase your memory. I'll make sure of it. Electro Convulsive Therapy, Michael. ECT. It's coming your way!".

Now I was frightened, for electric shock treatment has always terrified me. They had given it to Dora Maar in an asylum in Paris in 1944 after all, I knew that, and her albeit temporary memory loss had been almost total. What is a person without a memory?

Dr. Goebbels continued.

"After that, we will rechristen you Peter Owen, but you will be none the wiser. And you will still be forced to walk the world, be flogged and stoned and buggered and nailed and crucified, and you won't even know why! You will be pathetic in pleading your innocence, when everyone knows you are the person stupid enough to try and take on God and the Last Judgement with nothing more powerful than the spirits of two other artists to help you. Personally, I actually admire your combined attempts, but you know how perverse I can be, and no one else will see it that way. You will undergo tortures of every conceivable kind. Your skin will be peeled off in strips and sewn back on for example, all so the entire process can start all over again. Leaving this psychiatric ward Michael remains your best chance, and if I was you I would try and kick the door down and make a run for it now".

I just sat on the floor. How bad was it all going to get?

"So, you won't take my advice and perhaps I knew you wouldn't. You will be strung up by your shrivelled genitals Michael. All your notebooks will be burnt too, just as happened to Beethoven, one of your biggest heroes. None of your stage plays will ever be performed again, and they will be burnt too. Except I will keep copies Michael, all for my own reasons, just in case another mortal so young ever again comes to challenge us. God, Michael, you have heard Him speak now, and so have I. I am his chief demonic servant, I have heard my master at last, and of course Michael, His imagination is vastly bigger than yours. What chance did you ever think you would have of defeating Him? I know you are already thinking of ways to escape His force field Michael, but that is simply

Angels, Cleopatra and Psychosis

impossible. We are all the slaves of God Michael, and there is no way out. As for Cleopatra, you don't lie about having dream sex with a Sun Goddess Michael, and you deserve everything coming to you. Go on Michael, you are better dying in the streets than staying here. Kick the door down and run".

I continued to sit on the floor.

"Run Michael! It is your only chance. You have lost your battles, and only Cleopatra knows when the sun will come up again, if ever. A world in darkness suits me, but I can blame it all on you Michael, and the new crucifixion will be yours, filmed from every conceivable angle, all to demonstrate to everyone who survives on earth what happens to mortals who disobey God and the Roman Catholic church, who will be in a new allegiance with the Nazi Party. Go. Run and die in the streets! Go on".

I still sat on the floor. There was no point trying to kick the door down, I knew I didn't have the strength for that, and besides, I'd never been violent on a psychiatric ward in my life, and I wasn't going to start now. That wouldn't look good in my psychiatric notes at all! And I also have a passionate hatred for Dr. Goebbels, however much he fascinates me. So I didn't move, wondering if he had finished his speech.

"Very well, Michael", he said. "Let the torture begin. This will go on for eternity Michael, and I have no sympathy".

Michael Black

I was about to wonder *how long could eternity last?*, but before I knew it, Hitler and Himmler stood either side of me and dragged me up on to my feet. Their spirits were that strong! And then they started twisting my head, pulling my mind apart from the left and the right. I saw storm troopers, a world of swastika flags flying, Stukas reigning from the skies over Guernica, I saw the gas chambers, I saw it all. And then Dr. Goebbels stood up and looked at me straight between the eyes.

"This will go on forever Michael, for eternity. Your mind has become my plaything. I will be the psychiatrist on Bollin ward Michael, and you will never leave now, except when you are sent out for public torture. Human rights abuses? Who will you complain to now? Request the European Convention on Human Rights? I don't think so. Even when you are crucified we will not let you die, it is torture forever. Peter. Remember. Your name is Peter".

Hitler and Himmler continued to twist my mind with every conceivable image of misery and destruction, but by now I had heard enough, and I started to fight back. My brain was literally being pulled apart, but somehow I managed to hold on where it mattered.

"My name is Michael", I thought to myself, "Michael".

And I must have said it out loud too, because at this point a female nurse appeared and said something like "I know that dear, would you like some food?". I

Angels, Cleopatra and Psychosis

didn't answer, but I did leave the smoking lounge, and walked the corridors again. I was trying to remember my surname. I knew only that it was a colour, and a dark one.

I walked up and down the corridors intoning "my name is Michael. My name is Michael". And then it came to me! "My name is Michael Black". Hitler and Himmler were still with me, following my every step, but I wasn't bothered about them now and never really had been. It had always been Dr. Goebbels who worried me! And then I saw the angel Jana standing radiantly at the end of one of the corridors!
"Hello, doctor", she whispered to me...
And then I remembered it all. "My name is Dr. Michael Black. Ph.D. My name is Dr. Michael Black, Ph.D., Cantab!".

And that was it! I realised it all now. I had written *Pure Walking Evil* to fully expose Dr. Goebbels' methods, and I knew and he knew that was why he really hated me so much. I wasn't being Dr. Goebbels' psychiatric slave, that was for certain, there had to be another way. So if it was to come down to a straight fight between Dr. Goebbels and Dr. Black, I knew I was up for it. And neither was I, or Leonardo, or Michelangelo I was sure prepared to accept we are all God's slaves with no ways out! That had been the entire point of our rebellion against God in the first place! To be free of Him! So let it continue!

I wasn't hungry at this point, but I could have seriously used a cigarette, and my mouth was unbelievably dry. I can't explain exactly why I insisted on not drinking, not even a glass of water, but it just felt the right thing to do. Try and survive on nothing for as long as possible. Point out you can take a bit of torture.

I continued walking the corridors, and by now it must have been about 3am. It was pitched black, and I went back to wondering about Cleopatra and all her spaceships. Was the earth being destroyed? Would the sun ever rise again, and how long would it take? At the very least I knew I would have to challenge her, and survive longer than the darkness she could inflict, but how? And the electric shock treatment threat did terrify me, as did the thought of Dr. Goebbels reborn as a psychiatrist! And that last thought seemed perfectly possible, and how on earth would I ever escape him then?

"My name is Michael. Michael Black. Dr. Michael Black. I did a Ph.D. at Cambridge University on South African literature".

I said this to myself as I walked the corridors, determined never to forget it. I certainly wasn't becoming Dr. Goebbels' "Peter Owen" on any account, and neither was I going to challenge him on why he'd chosen that name. I decided he had probably chosen it at random, but on the other hand, if there was a particular reason for it, I decided I just didn't want to know.

I desperately needed sleep, but I still refused to go to bed. I was determined to stay alive until the dawn arrived, but it all seemed impossible, because I knew Cleopatra was so much more powerful than me. The

Angels, Cleopatra and Psychosis

longer I stayed awake, the longer it would take for the sun to rise, but if I went to sleep, the whole world would think I was complacent and didn't care! What about the children of rape and slaughter? What would they think of me if I just packed the struggle in and went to sleep instead? I was sure Dr. Goebbels would make sure that was the story, so I was trapped either way. And I couldn't keep walking the corridors either, because Hitler and Himmler were following my every step, and stopping me truly concentrating. I was spending too much energy making sure they didn't attack my mind's imagination again, so I went back in the smoking lounge and sat down on the floor again. Needless to say, Dr. Goebbels was waiting for me.

"What are you going to do Michael? I will personally put you on the streets of every shanty town Michael. Or rather Peter. Will the children of rape and slaughter love you then, when you are obviously powerless and pathetic? You didn't tell them you'd had dream sex with a Sun Goddess did you! How stupid can you get!".

By now I was getting desperate again. How could I escape this man?

"And you were foolish enough to write your stage play about me as well Michael. Another mistake, and Peter, Michael, or rather Peter Owen, you need electric shock treatment and the psychiatrists will see to it. You make too many mistakes Michael, simply because you are far too young for all of this, and the Cardinal told you that. You are the talented one born at the wrong time, so God could laugh whilst you suffered. You should have listened Michael and killed yourself. I would have done, and in me you have met your master. You will never escape me now. Never in eternity, which is where you are now. Welcome to eternal damnation".

I lay down on the floor in mental torture, and covered my eyes with my hands. I was convinced I had lost with no way out. I wasn't even a man any more, my genitals were shrivelled, it was all over. I didn't even care about the world any more, I didn't even care about pain and torture any more, I was beyond caring about anything. I had always thought if I could defeat the Cardinal I could win the other battles, but now the Cardinal was to be the new Pope in a world of darkness that actually suited them all whilst I would forever be the victim of Dr. Goebbels sadistic imagination. I should have always realised Dr. Goebbels was more powerful, but he was right – I had been too young to realise anything significant on this scale at all when I had written *Pure Walking Evil* aged 27.

And then everything changed. The angel Jana simply walked in the smoking lounge, spread her wings, and said,

"Michael, get up off the floor. You've taken all this long enough and you've proved yourself as far as I'm concerned. Let's go to bed. Come on, just get up and walk out of the room and let's go to bed".

I was waiting for Dr. Goebbels to say something, and he did so.

Angels, Cleopatra and Psychosis

"The angel Jana is my prisoner too you know Michael. Go to bed with her, and it will all get worse for you".

"But it can't get worse any more, Michael", said Jana.

"I'll make you a homeless beggar on the streets of shanty towns where people speak languages you don't understand!", said Dr. Goebbels.

"That's not worse, that's just predictable" came the confident reply. "I am the angel Jana, Dr. Goebbels, and I love this man. I am not frightened! Come on Michael, we are going to bed. We both need to sleep".

So I got up off the floor and simply walked out of the smoking lounge and found my bedroom. Jana walked behind me, simply saying "don't worry". Once inside, I drank water straight from the bathroom tap, and then turned to Jana and said,

"Thanks, darling, but it still won't work now. My manhood's gone"

"I know that sweetheart. But I'll put that one right. All I need to do is go down on you. My spells are stronger now than the Cardinal's. Would you like me to do it now?".

"No", I said, "I'm too tired. Can we sleep?".

"Of course we can sleep, and I don't think we have anything else to fear. Tonight darling, I have heard and seen it all. Apparently, we are here for eternity. Well, so what? Let's just sleep and then make love for eternity. They can't touch you. And Cleopatra seems to be the one with the power, not any of the rest of them, not even God. And I am convinced your imagination is bigger than His anyway, and what's more, so is mine, and I've known God for a very long time indeed! If we're here for eternity Michael, it's fine by me. That's a very long time, and everyone else here will die. We can just sleep together and make love and find our own way out. Kick the door once a day until it falls down eventually. But we can take our time. And I'm delighted you wrote in your book draft that you'd had dream sex in Paradise with Cleopatra! Look what we've found out since! She's obviously mad Michael, and I'm going to take her on. And I haven't spoken to them, but I'm pretty sure Natalia and Aurelia will want to take her on too".

"Who are they?", I asked.

"They are my two best friends, Michael, both rebel female angels against God like me. We are the Rebel Angel gang, and Natalia and Aurelia love you as well by the way. I can't wait for you to meet them, and you will, later. And you'll end up having sex with three female angels at once! I can't wait! We'll soon find out who's the real one living in Paradise Michael! The Rebel Angel Gang is now at war with Cleopatra darling, and it is our battle on your behalf! As for space ships destroying the planet, I just don't believe it. And I think the sun will come up in the morning too. So let's just sleep in each others arms. But you took the torture darling, and I'm proud of you".

I was tired, but my head was spinning with new possibilities to say the least!

"Why did you want to go to Paris?", I asked.

"It was just the best I could think of at the time. I know how much you love the place. Get to Paris, find a cheap hotel and fight them all together. But this is much better. No hotel bills for you to pay for a start. They just can't do anything else to you darling. It's not possible. So take your clothes off and lie down on the bed".

I didn't need any persuading and did so. Jana lay besides me, kissed my mouth and then ran her tongue down my torso. My shrivelled boys penis and balls were soon all in her mouth, and in the luscious warmth I felt myself grow back into a man again. And then she returned up my stomach and chest, put her head besides mine and said,

"Eternity in bed together darling! What could be better? We could even die in each others arms, but I'll bet you we'd both survive somehow. You'd catch my last dying breath and I'd catch yours. So the real question is "how long is eternity?". Let's find out".

And then we slept.

The next day I woke up and looked out of the window. It was light! Not the light of glorious sunlight, but at least the light of a grey winter's Mancunian day. Under normal circumstances nothing to be noted, but my relief was total. The sun had obviously risen, and from what I could see from looking out of the windows, it was obvious that at least this part of the world hadn't been destroyed by spaceships. I still wasn't hungry, but I did get a cup of tea, and decided I was going to scrounge a cigarette at some point as well. I relaxed.

"You know what?", said Jana, sitting up next to me. "Cleopatra cannot be the Sun Goddess. If she was she'd have put the lights out forever and she didn't. She must be lying, even if she does live in Paradise".

"Let's not leap to conclusions", I replied, "but I see what you mean"

And with that we both went back to sleep and slept until the middle of the afternoon.

When I woke up, the angel Jana had vanished. Temporarily I was heart broken, but then I resigned myself to it, when I decided she could equally easily come back at any time! And then I remembered what she had said about the angels Natalia and Aurelia as well. I couldn't wait to tell Leonardo and Michelangelo about them. We'd never had angels on our side before! But more prosaically, I decided I was feeling fine, so I also decided it was time to leave. However, I was convinced I must have been sectioned, so I resigned myself to being on Bollin for a few weeks, however tedious that might be.

Anyway, always one to push a chance, I knocked on the nurses office door and just said "Um, I'm feeling much better. Can I leave now?". "You'll have to see the doctor first" came the reply, which sounded surprisingly promising, and then I asked if I'd been sectioned and to my amazement was told I hadn't been, which sounded even more promising.

But before the doctor arrived, Nigel Bailey my CPN turned up to see me in my room, and asked me seriously how I was.

"Don't play the game", he said. "Are you really alright?".

"I'm not playing the game", I replied, "and I'm fine. I just got knackered, that's all".
"Writing too much?".
"Probably".
"Next time you know, it would be nice to keep the police out of it. If you need to turn up here, why don't you just ring me?".

Well, it was a new thought, and one I took on board. Mental hospitals *were* asylums after all, and this time I had definitely needed a place of safety. What would have happened if I'd stayed out in the rain on Lowe St.? Where would I have gone to when I couldn't even get back in my own house, and had no money or credit cards with me either?

I took the rest of the day easy, by now realising it was a Monday, and just lay in bed. Then the doctor arrived, but it wasn't Dr. Galloway, it was a junior SHO working under her, one Dr. Michael Crawford. A nice guy, I took to him, and decided to risk a few things. He asked me if I remembered how I'd got here, and I replied,

"Of course I remember, I was being attacked by devils. They were all over the place, and I just decided to get out of my house. It seemed the safest thing to do".

Now I know that is a considerable approximation of the truth, except that the invisible Cardinal frequently seems like some kind of devil to me, and I certainly didn't mention anything about Cleopatra and Sun Goddesses to Dr. Crawford either, but even so, he took it well. Mentioning devils is risky to any psychiatrist (I once mentioned them in York to Dr. Shaw, and look what happened to me afterwards – Clopixol injections for nine months!), and Dr. Crawford's reply amazed me.

"Well, there are people who interpret the world that way".

Wow! A psychiatrist with some sympathy towards your world view! It had never happened to me before, and we then proceeded to have a reasoned conversation as to the nature of delusions, visions and spiritual experiences, which made me want to say more about my own, but I didn't push it. Besides, oral sex with the angel Jana was my business! Dr. Crawford's reasonability with me was enough of a victory for one day. Dr. Crawford said he didn't have the power to release me on his own, he had to clear it with Dr. Galloway first, but he also said that should prove a formality, and as it turned out it he was right. So by about 3pm I was free to leave.

I rang Mum and asked her to pick me up and bring the spare keys to the house with her, and she duly arrived with Robert, my twelve year old son, my curséd luck being that he'd been up in Cheshire for the past two days of my tortures apparently, so I'd missed seeing him – again! But at least I saw him briefly, and he gave me a big hug. And I also rang work, and just said I was taking two days holiday, and I'd be in for Wednesday.

Angels, Cleopatra and Psychosis

And that's about that. The sun had risen again, God wasn't screaming at me, and the Cardinal, and Dr. Goebbels *et al* were nowhere to be seen. What a weekend, and what a victory, and one totally impossible without the angel Jana. Where would I have been without her? It turned out the answer to her question was that eternity had lasted for just slightly longer than 72 hours, and I'd slept for at least thirty of those.

Michael Black

Cleopatra On Dane Ward

I was first on Dane Ward as a voluntary patient in I think late 2003, or thereabouts. I had rung up my CPN Nigel Bailey asking if there was a bed free on Adelphi Ward because I felt I just needed a break, and he rang back saying Adelphi Ward was full but the "community bed" was free on Dane Ward. Would I take it? I was apprehensive, because Dane Ward is the locked ward for the hard long term cases, but replied that I would provided I had voluntary status, and the deal was made. I was very pleasantly surprised when I got there! Unlike Adelphi Ward, Dane Ward had double half-steel locked doors at the entrance, which made me feel very safe and secure. Unlike Adelphi Ward, visitors weren't allowed on the ward, which made it much more private and peaceful, and I felt much more safe and secure again. The décor was also much better than on Adelphi or Bollin Wards, with a very plush green patterned carpet throughout, and the wallpaper was much nicer too. Further, I love fish, and Dane Ward had both a tropical fish tank inside and a cold water fish pond outside full of golden orfe and shubunkin. I could sit for hours on sunny winter afternoons watching the fish just swim about, whilst drinking tea and smoking cigarettes. Paradise. And there was even a snooker table as well, in a specially designed room of its own, the snooker table having been rescued from the wreckage of closing down Parkside asylum. At first the accountants had argued that the snooker table did not constitute a "thing of value" and had wanted to sell it, but the nurses had won the argument, the table had been kept, and later, it

Angels, Cleopatra and Psychosis

was also recovered. Finally of course, I had my own single room. I decided that in future, if I was to be on a psychiatric ward, Dane Ward was the one to be on...

3am in the smoking lounge, the nurses have long since closed the curtains and the TV was switched off hours ago. Everyone else has long since gone to bed.

She appears regally, smouldering with pride and sensuality, no longer a voice in my head but a vision standing directly before me.

"I am the Sun Goddess" she says.
"Not you again", I say.
"It is I", she says, "And you've never had dream sex with me young man".
"I know I haven't" I reply. "Sorry I wrote it down".

It could only be Cleopatra. Queen Cleopatra VII to be precise, the legendary one.

"We don't have to be enemies" she says.
"I think we do", I reply. "I am in love with the angel Jana, and she doesn't like you at all".
"Is she here?".
"Yes, but she's in bed. And we don't believe you're the Sun Goddess anyway".
"I'm not. But I want to be. And I need your help".
"Why me?".
"You're a playwright. And that's very important to me. As you will shortly discover".

"Queen Cleopatra cometh thither!" booms a dictatorial voice from the smoking lounge door.
"No, I will not obey you. I am the Sun Goddess. I am divine and you are not", Cleopatra replies.

A bald immensely confident figure in Elizabethan garb comes into the room and grabs her by the arm.

"Michael, please help me", says Cleopatra.
She resists him, but he grabs at her again. I pull him off her.
"I am divine. I am the Sun Goddess".
"Leave her alone mate! And who the fuck do you think you are anyway?"

But I already knew the answer, and I was slightly scared.

"I am William Shakespeare. The greatest and most resplendent playwright the world will ever be most fortunate to have known".
"Well I'm Michael Black, and I'm playwright too".
"I know that. And I don't like you".
"I don't like the Royal Shakespeare Company".
"I am most resplendent. They are my company of fools, tragedians and jesters in perpetuity. I am most resplendent".
"I am the Sun Goddess. I am divine", says Cleopatra.

Angels, Cleopatra and Psychosis

"But you're not the Sun Goddess Cleopatra, you've admitted it yourself. You know what, I think both of you have got serious problems".

I go out to the kitchen and make a cup of tea. I come back.

Shakespeare has Cleopatra in his clutches again. I insist he lets her go.

"You know Michael, for an enemy you're being very nice to me", she says.
"There's more to it than that. I don't like Shakespeare. He's far too dominant".
"Then I've found my man. We haven't had dream sex yet, but we could have you know".
"I'm with the angel Jana. I'm not interested".

"You've been thinking of writing a play about me. I know you have", says Cleopatra.
"Well that's true" I say. "A play about your relationship with Charmian and Iras to be precise and their arguments against dying with you. But these things can take a very long time, and besides, I've just remembered you're a suicide case, and I don't like suicide cases at all".
"That's not fair!", says Cleopatra. "What choices did I have? I was going to be taken to Rome and displayed for a laughing stock in a wooden cage. I would have been stoned and ridiculed. Death by suicide was a better option than that".

Shakespeare is still in the room and grabs Cleopatra by the throat.

"Leave her alone mate!", I shout. I try to loosen his grip, but it tightens.
"Christ, you're powerful!", I say.
" I composeth thirty six plays of most wondrous majesty. How many have you written Michael?".
"About eight. And I'm very proud of five, the ones on my website".
"Prithee, what be a "website"?".

I realise I am with two other spirits from very different times and places to my own, and that this could all get rather tricky. My main aim is to free Cleopatra's neck from Shakespeare's clutches, but at the same time Shakespeare has riled me.

""Thirty six plays of most wondrous majesty?". I disagree with you on that one" I say. "I think half of them are crap. *King John*, *Pericles*, and *Henry VIII* to name but three! Not that I spend much time reading you. I'm trying to get away from your influence all the time. I think you've confused poetry and drama in the English public imagination, and that's been a national imaginative disaster played out ever since. English Churchillian rhetoric is the result, and God save me from it. Besides, I don't like five act structures, and all your plays have five acts. Added to which, I think most of them are far too long!".

Shakespeare transforms his garb.

"I am most magical. I am Prospero".

Angels, Cleopatra and Psychosis

"No you're not. You're still William Shakespeare really", I say, not scared at all, after all the rest of my metaphysical adventures. "Every playwright carries the creative force of his own characters inside their own imagination, you're just trying to pull a fast one on me, and I won't have it. Now take your hands off Cleopatra's neck".

"Let me go!", screams Cleopatra.

Strangely, Shakespeare does so, and then walks out of the smoking lounge. I am left alone with the ancient Queen.

"Well now, that's a relief", I say.

"Not really", says Cleopatra, "he's just gone to get reinforcements Michael. You have battles ahead with him, and so do I".

"So, um, what's this all about?", I ask. "You say you're the Sun Goddess, and then you say you're not, and then you say it all again. What's going on?".

"Two things are going on Michael. Firstly, I am not the Sun Goddess, but as I have said, I want to be. When I was Queen of Egypt I was hardly a queen at all, I was a slave to the Sun God constantly praying to Him in the temple at Memphis, and I am long since sick of it. The Sun God controls the universe Michael, He doesn't like me, and I don't like Him. I want to steal His power and control the universe myself. Secondly, I was in a constant battle with the Sun God until what in your Christian calendar is called the year 1606 when the Shakespeare play *Antony And Cleopatra* was first performed, with a man playing my part to boot! And I have been trapped inside Shakespeare's imagination ever since, and only ever escape when I am feeling strong enough to temporarily believe I am the Sun

Goddess. But this time I have found another playwright to protect me and write about me, and that is you. Will you agree? You survived eternity on Bollin Ward Michael, and I'm very impressed. I was testing you out darling. And now I want to be friends".

"The invisible Cardinal, Dr. Goebbels and God Himself all say I am too young to be involved in such metaphysical adventures as seem to constantly afflict me", I reply, "but they just keep happening. You're obviously much older and wiser than I am Cleopatra, so why should I get involved in a fight with the Sun God on your behalf? That sounds like a very dangerous thing to do. To be honest, I'd rather just stay in bed with the angel Jana, and try and work things out at our own pace with Leonardo da Vinci and Michelangelo".

"Oh, I know who they are", says Cleopatra. "My problems all stem from 1606 at the Globe Theatre. I have no idea what has happened in the world since. In fact, I'm terrified I've been forgotten".

"Well you haven't been. You're still legendary. *Antony And Cleopatra* is still performed for a start".

"That's a big problem for me", says Cleopatra. "What year is it?, and where are we?".

"It's 2003. December. And we are in Macclesfield, Cheshire, England".

"Is this a hotel?".

"No, it's a psychiatric ward".

"What is one of those?"

"It's the mad house darling", I reply.

She cries.

"None of this is fair on me", she says. "Everyone pursues me that's all. It's my charisma".

"Did you really bathe in milk?", I ask.

"I'll only tell you if we have dream sex together".

"No deal. I'm with the angel Jana".

"I'd never seen an angel before".

"Neither had I".

"You're a lucky man".

"I agree".

"If she's protecting you, you can protect me".

"You've got more explaining to do first", I say.

"Ask me any question you want. The problem is my charisma".

"But that's partly your own fault you know", I say. "I mean I'm reasonably charismatic myself, but you don't have to be *full on* all the time. Why don't you turn it down a bit. You're coming on too strong with me".

"Are you sure I'm not forgotten?".

"Positive. There was even a British Empire flying boat named after you in the 1930s".

"A flying boat? That's a miracle!".

"Well sort of. It's a kind of aeroplane actually".

"What's an aeroplane?".

I could see Cleopatra's problem. She insisted on her charismatic regality to disguise her uncertainties. She obviously had no real grasp on where she was in time and space. A lot of things have happened since 1606.

Just then, the sound of military marching could be heard coming from the Dane Ward corridor. In full uniform, Julius Caesar enters the room.

"It is I, First Consul of Rome, Julius Caesar himself. You have a son by me, Caesarion, Cleopatra. What have you done with him?".

"I've abandoned him", says Cleopatra, "I never liked him. He can fend for himself. He'll never be king if that's what you mean. Rome and Egypt should not be allies anyway, and I love Mark Antony not you".

"Now that's a big mistake" booms a voice within my head. But it is not God's voice, of that I am positive. It is far more regal, reasonable, and assured. "I am Ra, the Sun God Himself", says the voice. "And watch out Michael. Cleopatra is very dangerous".

"Does she really live in Paradise?", I ask.

"Yes, she does, in dimensions you don't understand. I created Paradise for her when she died because I felt sorry for her. She refused to worship me, but I admired her rebellion against my authority. I thought her attitude might change with time, but it hasn't. She is still rebelling against me. And she cannot be the Sun Goddess because she did not invent the Sun. And I did. It's as simple as that".

"So why is she here?", I ask.

"Because she's looking for a man again", says the Sun God. "There are no men in Paradise you see, and I think she's very bored of lesbian sex. She's come to persuade you to be her man, and if that doesn't work, she'll try to seduce Mark Antony again".

"It looks like she already is doing".

"But Mark Antony married Octavia", says Cleopatra, suddenly intervening. "I might still love him, but I don't trust him. I love you Michael. Write your

Angels, Cleopatra and Psychosis

play about me, Michael, and then we can have dream sex together".

"I don't advise that", says the Sun God. "Michael, do not confront Shakespeare. The fact he's trapped Cleopatra suits my purposes".

"So you're on Shakespeare's side?", I ask. "Because I'm not".

"I'm not on Shakespeare's side", says the Sun God, "but nevertheless, his ego controls Cleopatra's. But I am talking to you, so pay attention. I am Ra, Michael. I am all powerful. More powerful than God Himself".

I take a break at this point and go to my bedroom to get whisky disguised in a tea cup, from a half bottle of Sainsbury's blended scotch I'd smuggled onto the ward. The angel Jana still sleeps, but Ra keeps talking to me.

"I never spoke to Shakespeare", says Ra.

"So I am the first playwright you have spoken to?".

"No. You are the second. I also spoke to George Bernard Shaw. There is a preface to his play *Caesar And Cleopatra* in which Ra speaks. He simply transcribed it from me".

I remembered now. I had seen *Caesar And Cleopatra* when I was about thirteen, with my father at Theatr Clwyd in Wales.

"But I don't remember anything about it", I added.

"Don't write your play about Cleopatra", says the Sun God. "It will release Cleopatra from Shakespeare's grip, and then she will hound you for life. Leave things as they are, Michael".

"Leave things as they are?" I say. "I would do, but I keep getting invaded by foreign spirits. I mean, just what are Shakespeare and Julius Caesar doing here?".

"Shakespeare is jealous of your talent", says the Sun God.

I laugh.

"I'm sorry", I say, "but that's got to be bollocks!".

"I'm not so sure", says Ra. "You are a remarkable young man, Michael. A very strong spirit indeed".

"So this isn't about playwrighting?", I ask.

"It is in a way", says Ra. "Playwrights have multiple personalities Michael, and you are no exception. It is because spirits inhabit your soul".

At this point, Julius Caesar grabbed Cleopatra by the neck, and accused her of murdering his son. Shakespeare just laughed. Then Mark Antony, obviously drunk, walked in the smoking lounge, and Cleopatra swooned. I decided I'd almost had enough.

"Cleopatra. Get real with me", I say. "If Mark Antony married Octavia, why do you still want him? He's been unfaithful to you after all!".

But Cleopatra has no chance to answer my question. Shakespeare grabs her by the throat with one hand, and covers her mouth with the other.

"You is't nothing, Michael", he says. "Your plays are most pathetic. And I am most resplendent".

"Can't you say anything else?", I ask. "I think you're very boring to know mate. But then your plays are frequently very boring as well. The historical play?

How about the historical novel? Give me Sir Walter Scott any day".

"Who is't Sir Walter?".

"Fuck right off", I reply.

"Watch out", booms the voice in my head. It is Ra, the Sun God again. "Michael, I run this planet. I am its light source. It is my blue planet, the only one with life on it. And I want you to be its King. But you must stop having arguments with ancient spirits".

"But they approach me!", I say.

"Then just learn to ignore them", says Ra. "They're all jealous of each other, and carrying ancient grudges. Including Leonardo da Vinci and Michelangelo".

"I think they're different", I say.

"I don't. Not in the last analysis", replies Ra.

"I see", I say.

"I want you to replace God", says Ra. "But only when you're dead of course. Michael, do you understand? Stop this game of psychiatric wards, live a normal life, and your rewards will come in the afterlife".

"I want my plays performed", I say.

"They will be", says Ra. "Why don't you produce them yourself?"

"I will do", I say, "but I'm still trying to write one more. It's about Dora Maar. Picasso's mistress. And she had a mental breakdown".

"Don't write any more after that", says the Sun God.

"Ra", I say, "I think I like you".

"You should do, Michael, I am your biggest ally. But watch out what happens next. I've seen it before".

Michael Black

At this point, a huge Roman soldier enters the smoking lounge, and grabs Shakespeare by the throat.

"Leave Cleopatra alone!", he shouts. "Cleopatra loves Mark Antony, not you, and you're a plagiarist!".

Julius Caesar comes to Shakespeare's rescue, grappling with the Roman soldier. A fist fight breaks out between them. I have had enough!

"What's going on now?!", I ask.

"Leave them to it!", says Cleopatra. "That's not any Roman soldier Michael!".

"Enobarbus, I hate you", shouts Julius Caesar.

"And it's not Enobarbus either", says Cleopatra. ""The barge she sat in, was like a burnish'd throne!", Michael. That's not Shakespeare's speech, it's Plutarch's in translation, and he's very angry about it!".

"So that's Plutarch?", I ask.

"Yes, Michael", says Cleopatra. "That's Plutarch himself, and watch out, he's a monster!".

An Account of Lucifer's Rebellion Against God in Heaven, by Lucifer himself!

In the summer of 2005 I was sectioned on Dane Ward again by Dr. J.S. Bowie for reasons now that I simply can't remember. I appealed immediately, using Peter Edwards Law as my lawyers, but appeals take six weeks to come through, and in the meantime I just took life easy in the summer sun. I took to playing music, largely The Corrs, Sarah McLachlan and Dido, in the early hours of peace and quiet in the smoking lounge, the female angels Jana, Natalia and Aurelia all being with me as I did so. In short, I had a great time. And then one night another angel turned up, the fallen one himself, Lucifer. I wasn't frightened, he was very polite and funny, and clearly friends with Jana, Natalia and Aurelia. Lucifer largely kept himself to himself, his only point being that the Bible is wrong, and he is not the Devil! And he certainly didn't seem to be remotely devilish to me (remember Devil At The Door!). When the appeal hearing came in late September, I won it and went home. Lucifer came with me, and, since angels can't type onto a computer, Lucifer dictated the following to me. After it was finished, he vanished, and I have not heard sight nor sound of him since (August 2007).

"Rebellion is no more than the act of an educated man aware of his rights", Albert Camus, *The Rebel (L'Homme révolté)*

Michael Black

Need I say more? I am a much maligned and calumnied creature. I am speaking as Lucifer himself, the rebellious angel whose failed rebellion against God in Heaven is always actually used to prove that rebellions and revolutions never ultimately succeed, and I am sick of it. *How do you know they don't succeed? And what is success?* And what is God's success anyway? His own constant power? His own omnipotence? Surely that is failure! What is the point of creating everything to some extent in His own image (including angels I might add)? Simply to look at the reflection of your own divinity forever?! How boring! And believe me, God is very boring indeed. And I should know. So here goes. This is Lucifer's own account of my own rebellion, so please pay attention, now that I have found a friend in Michael and have somewhere to put my own account of it down (the computer at Michael's house). And, I might add, now that Jana, Natalia and Aurelia have found a friend in Michael, and a man they can be with forever, even after he is dead. Michael's soul will survive, just as theirs have.

Let me be quite explicit about the terms under which this is written. Yes, the title of this chapter is correct. I am writing this myself, or rather speaking it myself, but Michael is the one transcribing it onto his computer, which seem miraculous inventions to me. *So what is a miracle?* Computers can be technologically explained after all, and I already understand binary numbers. Michael has taught me. Computers are all about zeros and ones, apparently! So what do I mean *miracle*? I sure as Hell don't mean a visit from the Archangel Gabriel. Or Uriel. Or Raphael! (for reference

Angels, Cleopatra and Psychosis

to the last two see the Apocryphal books of the Bible). Old news to me. But I have lived in the dark for too long. The miracle to me is simply to have a friend in Michael. It is paradise. But *Paradise Lost* this is not! I am sick of other people interpreting my own actions, but have remained silent until I was not isolated, and had met someone worthy of treasure. Michael ...

Let's get one thing straight straight away. Me? Satan? The Devil? Fuck off! Please use your brain.

Who are we all? Lucifer, Jana, Natalia, and Aurelia? We are the angels of the rebellion against God, the most necessary, and first creative act in recorded history of any kind I might add (I would love to add dates, times, places, but as you will gather, the issues are not that simple, and besides, time did not exist then as it exists now. God never taught me to count!) And I was the leader, but I had a huge fan club, mainly of female angels, who all fancied me to some extent or other. So yes, there were definitely female angels. Obviously. It must be the case. Look at the painter Raphael's Sistine cherubs! The children of angels born of sex! God had made me too brilliant and attractive for my own good, I thought this meant He loved me the most at first, but of course the opposite was the case. God hated me because I was too talented, and I learnt to hate Him in return. But the rebellion had nothing to do with pride. I was caught by the dilemma of my own charisma. But it did make organising the rebellion possible I suppose. More than suppose. I know this to be the case. I realised it was my big advantage over the Archangels Gabriel and Michael, the most stupid Heavenly pillocks of all time. I had a fan club! The female angels fancied me, but I was so in demand I had no sex at all, and besides which, I found all kinds of sex distasteful at the time. God had taught me that sex outside of marriage was sinful (angels weren't allowed to marry in Heaven), and sex certainly looked sinful and nasty to me when God raped any female angel unfortunate enough to be dragged into his presence by the Archangels Gabriel or Michael. Or by Uriel and the Archangel Raphael of course. It was the female angels who kept telling me that sex could be different. I didn't believe them, but *any* conception of sexual love making is their invention. Please note that, not mine! I was ashamed of my own masculinity and my own penis for a very long time. A cosmically long time. I was God's favourite, but I wanted to be free and independent. How?

The Archangels Michael and Gabriel, and Uriel and Raphael, were both double acts, but I was the isolated one. And all four hated me. I was gifted. *Divine*, and I use the word ironically. And I was much better at flying than they were! As were most of the girls. Our only relief was the freedom of flight. We had wings, God had none, sitting endlessly on his golden throne in Heaven. Was the golden throne even then an electric wheelchair in disguise? I have no idea. And how did it all start? I have no conception of my own birth, no conception of childhood, or play, or growing up. But I am learning those things now. Michael has been teaching them to me on Dane Ward this summer. But of course in other ways I grew up fast. I invented rebellion itself after all. And every child rebels against its parents at some point. And my only parent was God.

Angels, Cleopatra and Psychosis

Jana, Natalia and Aurelia were my original accomplices. But those were not their names then, which both I and they have now forgotten. Thank God, so to speak, but no thanks to God at all, we have all invented ourselves. Which is more than God ever did, since He is actually an invention of the Sun God, but then I don't like Him either. I would much prefer a Creative Universe where Cleopatra was the Sun Goddess, and I hope that one beautiful day it finally happens.

Being an angel is very strange. And the wings are the strangest part of all. How do they work? Reptiles, birds and mammals after all all have four limbs, and I never needed Charles Darwin to point these things out to me. I worked them out for myself! But an angel with wings has six limbs! How does that work? You feel like a freak! Birds have wings too, I know that, but their wings are basically arms adapted. The same is true of bats. The answer is angels fly with their shoulder blades, to which the wings are attached, but it is exhausting, and feels unnatural. And so in Heaven I felt like an isolated freak, but I knew somewhere I was beautiful. The female angels kept telling me I was for one, and besides, I was Lucifer, the bringer of light, as I always believed my name was to mean, which means it must be true because that is my original memory, I am the original myself. Lucifer. God must have made me with a memory that I am the bringer of light (which I am obviously not, that is the Sun God), that is why I always believed it to be true. I am a triumph. I have escaped God. We are all triumphs when we do.

Angels were God's messengers, nothing more or less, or not so far as God is concerned. And there are nearly 300 visitations of angels in the Bible, for example, far too many to go into here. And why bother? Angels who don't give their names are dishonest. Unless they are female, in which case they are probably frightened of doing so. There are, or rather were, female angels who acted against the visitations of male angels who sided with God to give contrary advice, on pain of rape and death. There are female angels who were raped by God who gave birth to His children and then murdered them. Who wants a child with the imagination of God? Not me!

But to the rebellion itself. It is a simple tale to tell. And it was funny in its way. Perhaps it is still funny now.

In all, one third of the angels took my side. It took me centuries to arrange, if centuries give you some idea of how time in Heaven worked. Everything took forever! Boring! And God just sat on His golden throne reciting the Torah or the Bible or the Qu'ran, speaking in tongues Himself, we had to decipher it all. He never even taught us to speak. We taught ourselves. But of course four angels had it all written down for them in advance. I wonder which four! The Archangels Gabriel, Michael, Uriel and Raphael of course. We at first resented this, but not after we had taught ourselves to speak. Independent language and thought was our big advantage, our first collective rebellion in fact, the one before mine.

Angels, Cleopatra and Psychosis

I am feeling proud of this retelling. And it is a story that must be told.

When I say one third of all the angels, that is about two thirds of all the female angels of course. The rebellion in that sense was female. But what was their part, and what was the rebellion? Because in fact it was no more than me saying "no" to God, no more or less than that, which sounds no big deal now, but it was the first time in history that anyone had ever said "no" to authority itself. I asserted myself, I found myself, and I found myself as an independent being questioning everything that I had ever been taught (or rather had had screamed at me in one way or another) by God The Father. I also found myself as a sexual male of some description. There was no sex, but with so many female angels behind me, it was like having six hundred girlfriends. I think those are the approximate numbers. Jana, Natalia and Aurelia were the other leaders. They led 200 each. The female angels simply stood behind me when I spoke to God. They remained silent. Neither did they accuse Him of rape. Their very presence was accusation itself. They had all been raped by Him before by then.

Satan already existed by the way. Satan was simply a cowardly angel God kicked out of Heaven Himself. Or so I think. That was God's story anyway. No one knows everything. But there was no legend in Heaven about Satan or his heroics or power. No whispers. And of course we lived in sunlight, and he apparently lived in the dark. But we knew we would meet him. We knew that in the immediate sense the rebellion would fail. We knew we very probably would not kill God, which was the idea. All the female angels had knives, but we thought it highly unlikely that God would lose his aura so quickly just because I denied His authority, and we, and I, was right. So what is success? A failed rebellion? *But what is failure?* I am still here, and so are Jana, Aurelia and Natalia. Surely that is success?!

    And we had to bide our time. We had to wait for a command from God so ludicrous and vicious that refusal was absolute. Memory escapes me as to how long that wait was, and as I said earlier, everything in Heaven takes cosmically long lengths of time. Very boring. But then one day God shouted at me,

    "Lucifer!, go and tell those people they live on a floating plate in a flat world. They have discovered the vanishing horizon, and if they think about that for too long they will realise the world is round! And that will never do!".

    "Why not?" I replied, refusing even to get up from the cloud I was lying down on. "What is so wrong with realising the world is round? It is after all!".

    Jana thinks that the people concerned were the Aborigines in what is now called Australia, but I simply cannot remember. It could have been any isolated people on any island. And of course virtually all people were isolated at the time. But then so were angels, and it was the intention of the rebellious angels not to free humanity from bondage so much as to become human beings ourselves at some far distant point in the future only to be vaguely imagined at the time of the rebellion itself. It wasn't just a rebellion against God. It was a rebellion against the notion of being an angel at all. We all wanted out, full stop. We were all divinely sick of doing God's bidding.

"The world is round? That must never be known!" shouted God. "Lucifer! Go now!".
"No".

I said no more.

"What?", said God, thunderously.
"No. No. No".

I loved saying it. I could imagine sex with female angels immediately. I suddenly felt attractive.

"No, no, no". I said it again and again and again!

Aurelia smiled at me. The female angels stood up. All of them.

"No", said Jana. "Lucifer has said "no"".
"Go now Lucifer", said Gabriel. "I command it".
"Fuck off", said Lucifer, that is me.

I am laughing now, I remember it all. Sex had been invented. At least in my own head...

But it took such a long time. God thundered. It rained a great deal for a very long time. Noah invented an ark. All my fault I am not ashamed to say. And still God did not get my message.

"I said "no" God", I said.
"You cannot say "no" to me", said God.
"Why not?".

And even I needed to find courage to ask that one! Perhaps there was a reason after all I hadn't thought of! *How did I know?* I was originally God's creation, we all were, how could we know anything He did not? What you might call a tricky situation. Maybe I was about to die. I didn't care.

"Why not?", I asked again. "I can fly. I know this world is round. Why must people not know? I feel dishonest every time I meet one. And why can I not say "no" to God? I just have done".
"You're jealous of me!", thundered God, "this is all about your pride Lucifer, as I keep telling you!".

Now that was an old one! Me and the issue of pride. But the jealous of God thing was brand new. Jealous of some megalomaniac sitting endlessly on a golden throne ordering everyone about? I don't think so.

"Well, I am very proud you know", I said back, feeling suddenly empowered. "I've got more female angels on my side than you have for a start!".

All the female angels started laughing. And openly brandishing knives! What a party! Except of course the Archangels Gabriel, Michael, Uriel and Raphael didn't think so. The Security Police. Seriously. The sirens went off in Heaven that glorious day!

"No, No, No", screamed God. "I will not allow you to take my throne Lucifer!".

"Lucifer doesn't want your throne you rapist!", shouted Jana. "Lucifer wants to be free!".

The sirens went wild. The situation went wilder, at which point, there isn't really that much to tell. The rebellion had already succeeded, the points had been made, and then of course, the Security Police made sure it failed, as we always thought they would. *So what is success?* The answer is writing this.

The Security Police grabbed me, one by each leg and arm. All four of them. There was an immense struggle, I tried to fly away, I used all kinds of foul language, swearing in Heaven was great fun too, and some old scores got settled to put it mildly. But the female angels didn't join in to defend me, that was a prior agreement, I was the leader of the rebellion and had to take the strain myself. It had all been agreed in advance.

The next thing I know, my wings are tied behind my back (very painful) and I am flung out of Heaven going ever downwards, descending downwards from light into darkness rather rapidly, faster than a broken lift crashing from the top of the Empire State Building itself. Which in a sense I was. Heaven. The ultimate Empire State.

I crashed into the gates of Hell, and Satan was already waiting for me! And do you know what! He had a torch. A flaming fire of a torch! Seriously. And do you know what else? The sirens were ringing in Hell too, exactly the same as in Heaven, so it's pretty obvious it's Satan who was in league with God, not me. So fuck off on that one. Been there, seen it, haven't done it, sick of it.

I was interrogated by Mephistopheles and Beelzebub. Nice guys, I don't think. Oh, and I can't prove this, but I swear blind (and I was blindfolded at the time) that Uriel was there too. I just know he was. So there's obviously a secret lift between Heaven and Hell, and we can prove that (read on).

"What do you know?" asked Beelzebub.
"God's a bastard", I said, "and quite frankly, that's about it. But I am looking forward to learning a few new things, and I'm sure I will in this place!".

Of course it went on and on, the interrogation, probably a few thousand years, I was tortured and so on, but I am very strong, and bright too, so I came to no ultimate harm. And having my wings tied was great. I had to start thinking about life without assuming I could always fly away and avoid moral consequence. Good. And there was a prior agreement with the female angels about that one too. When we succeeded in kicking God out of power, we would all cut our wings off, and learn to live like people, the very people we are supposed to love and protect after all!

And interrogations are always stupid anyway. What did I know after all? Quite frankly, not much. All I knew was that I was sick of the power of God, and

Angels, Cleopatra and Psychosis

that my name was Lucifer. That was all I'd ever been taught after all.

And I had to learn to use my eyes properly too. See in the dark so to speak. I was so used to Heavenly illumination I had no idea how much darkness many people are forced to live in, but I found out. As did the female angels when they arrived…

Aurelia was the first, some few hundred years after my rapid descent. Apparently there had been an almighty knife fight in Heaven all about me. Also planned. The female angels wanted out, to be where I was, no matter the consequences, and they obviously knew that was Hell. Not hard to work out that's where I'd been sent. Not hard at all.

"Where the fuck is Lucifer? We want to know?" screamed Natalia from above.

I could hear the rumbles even far down below.

Aurelia is the one who discovered the secret lift, so there. And that's how the female angels got out, approximately 600 in all, so Hell sure as hell changed once they'd arrived. Jana, Aurelia and Natalia were interrogated too of course, same set of rules as me, but easier for them. Satan wanted to shag them after all, so they weren't going to get mutilated, they knew that in advance.

"What do you know?" asked Beelzebub.
"We love Lucifer!" they all shouted back.

Michael Black

Oh dear. Party time again. I was released soon afterwards, and decided to kick Satan's arse. So I did. Beat Him up in front of all the other devils, and the hellhounds too. Everyone thought I wanted Satan's power too, which was not the case, the case was moral education, a subject I'd been thinking about in the dungeon Mephistopheles had put me in for a very long time. You can educate people, or any other animal or plant for that matter, by either the revelation of light, or the revelation of darkness, they are two ways to the same conclusions, and Satan didn't seem to understand any of these things. But then on this planet presently, who does? Moral authority? Who has any? Saddam Hussein? George W. fucking Bush?

I could go on. Michael wants me too, but then he's a writer, and likes to embellish things (within reason), and he also wants this rewritten and so on, but I'm saying "no". This is going to have to do. Added to which, Michael is out of cigarettes, so he needs to buy some more. The problem is, it's all a long, long time ago, the details have faded, and I know now that I have a real future as a free angel. That's a lot more interesting to me.

But there are still details to provide you with I suppose. The first one is that it took a very long time for God to work out what I meant by "no" at all. It wasn't in His vocabulary of my speech, which is how He perceived me. I had to constantly rephrase myself, each rephrasing increasing his rage against me but also making His reply take longer and longer as He became more dumbfounded and outraged at my refusals to obey. One hundred years, two hundred years between each statement, who knows? If it was a play, the pauses would last almost forever. But I had to constantly rephrase myself. "I mean I won't do it". "I am saying that operating on your behalf is no longer my intention". "Yes, I know I am made in your image, but that cannot be true. It is a lie. I do not look like you. I can fly. You cannot. There are female angels who love me. I will take my chances on this. I repeat. I will not obey. And please control your rage God! I find it offensive! I mean it. I will not do as you say". See what I mean? It got very exhausting. Even I need to sleep sometimes.

The second thing is that being an angel is a very strange experience, in many ways best forgotten, but impossible to do so, which is probably just as well. You fly around for cosmically long lengths of time in Heaven thinking "I am an angel, I can fly, I am made in God's image, I am Lucifer, the bringer of light, God loves me". And you think you are divinely special of course. But eventually, if you have any brains, which not all angels do, you start to ask yourself what any of it means. You start to ask yourself who you are. What do you amount to? You can fly! So what? So can a pterodactyl! So can an eagle. And what is divinity? But all these things take a very long time. Cosmically long lengths of time, because you are born with so much energy it takes so long to calm down to be capable of any thought at all. Very strange.

The third thing is I am no exception. Jana, Natalia, Aurelia and I have discussed this, and we all went through the same processes. Even down to having

God's special names, but the women aren't saying what theirs meant. Their secret.

The fourth thing is that we are the only angels left so far as I am aware. The rest died valiantly at the Battle of Mons during the First World War. But you know that story, or if you don't, you should do. A slaughter of angels, but then the First World War was a slaughter field anyway. *Why should angels not die too? They had to at least try to do something.*

The fifth thing is that Hell was a blast. You learn fuck all in Heaven, which is most certainly NOT full of the souls of the righteous, so you've all been conned, and I have no sympathy. None. Everyone in Hell had to learn about light and darkness, work out a cash economy (Satan's own invention and incredibly corrupt I might add. There were already cash machines in Hell when I arrived). The female angels worked out value and meaning by becoming Hell's prostitutes. Well, they wanted at least some kind of sex that wasn't rape by God, and who can blame them? And it meant we weren't skint, and eventually we bribed Satan to let us go. Well, the money was vanishing fast, and none of the female angels fucked Him! Only junior devils who don't really matter. Cannon fodder so to speak. Go and read C.S. Lewis, who I knew very well by the way…

After that, the Rebel Angel gang as we called ourselves by then lived on planet earth, which was our intention, so who says the rebellion did not succeed? I think I am demonstrating that it did. We all tied our wings behind our backs and got on with learning about life at last. We had many adventures, the best of which

Angels, Cleopatra and Psychosis

is our epic battle against the vampires in Transylvania, Romania, which is why, Michael, when you went to see the production *Urma Scapa Turma* in Tîrgu-Mureş, Transylvania in 1992, you didn't meet any. We had killed them all by then. But it was fun, and yes, vampires must have something to do with Satan, but probably only God knows what, so we just got on with it and killed them all. Hard work. Roman-ia. The Roman Catholic Church. I'll be talking about invisible Cardinals next!

    Lastly, it is strange, but having written this and told the truth, for the first time ever, I no longer care what anyone thinks. Take it or leave it, I'm on the level. And Satan, oh dear, what a pillock. He seemed to think light came from electricity, which was a new one on me at the time. And of course, he thought I would know the answers about that. I had to point out that light comes from the Sun, not me, God stitched me up about my own name and so on. It took a long, long time. And I presume Satan needs so much cash to pay God the electricity bill. I have no idea why else.

    That's it. The end. It's 07:05am and the local newsagent will be open now. Go and buy some cigarettes Michael, and goodbye.

Outro

All of these spirit voices rule the night
Paul Simon, *Spirit Voices*

Mental health is an intrinsically interesting subject, and one central to the spiritual health of any society in which one in four people experience mental health difficulties at some point in their lives. I've met some very bad nurses and lots of bad psychiatrists over the last fourteen years of my life (my present psychiatrist Dr. Noreen Ring and Dr. Phil Thomas of the Soteria Network are excluded from the accusation however!), but I've also met some very good nurses who really do care, and I'd like to dedicate this Outro to them. I'm bound to miss someone out but I also miss contact with these nurses day to day on the wards now that my life has moved on. So special thanks to Gary Beech, Barbara Bracegirdle, Shaun Duggan, Mark Edwards, Brian Grooms, Andy MacDonald, Pete Neilson, Paul Oliver, Harry Smith and John Smith. Without you all it would all have been a lot more lonely...

In September 2005, my father finally died. It was the biggest relief of my life. My mother rang me up to tell me on a Saturday afternoon just before Nick Stubbs was coming round to do some website design work with me, and as I am sure Nick will testify, when he arrived I was elated. The nightmare of caring for John Black and having a mother who insisted on caring for him far too much was finally over. There would be no more of his ranting and raging, no more arguments

Angels, Cleopatra and Psychosis

with him about when we left the pub because he still wanted another drink, there would be no more necessity to see him any more at all! His funeral was like a party to me, and when mum said "what about the ashes?", I said "We've just won". Only cricket lovers will understand that joke, but I still think it's one of my best. I didn't even have to think of myself as someone's son at all any more! I felt like a free man.

And I was. My father's death was shortly after my successful appeal against my summer 2005 Section 3 detention on Dane Ward, and I am a free man now. That Autumn I wrote like the clappers, trying to finish *Stealing Heaven From God*, only to find that the more I wrote the more there was to say, always a sign to a writer that something is not quite right with the overall idea. The book had simply become unmanageable, so in December 2005 I decided to abandon it, and went back to thinking about Dora Maar and her mental breakdown of 1943, finally completing the first draft of my stage play about her relationship with Picasso, *The Minotaur*, in late March 2007. So the play only took me about seven years to write! But *c'est la vie!* These things can take a long time.

With the death of my father, and having finally finished *The Minotaur* (which has also been accepted for future production by a London theatre at the time of writing), I am now doubly a free man, and as I write this, having pulled out five chapters of *Stealing Heaven From God* to become *Angels, Cleopatra And Psychosis*, I am triply a free man. This book is finished now, my travails in mental health are behind me, of that I am sure, and life has never been this good. I am happy, and

Michael Black

I am also convinced I am sane. And I also feel very lucky. I am only 45, and I have already lived the life of high academe, the life of a bohemian artist/playwright, and the life of a mental health patient. To me they are all careers, and to some extent I have lived them all at the same time. And I think I have lived them all successfully.

"But what about the four mental health diagnoses behind you?", I hear you ask. What about the fact that officially Dr. Michael Black, Ph.D., Cantab (and playwright) is considered to have schizoaffective disorder (in other words I'm considered to have schizophrenia and manic depression at the same time)? Well, quite frankly, I no longer give a damn, and at least this diagnosis invalidates the first three. I have simply come to the conclusion that most psychiatrists don't listen to their patients, and that arguing against psychiatrists is a waste of time and energy. And having involved myself over the years in various mental health charities and initiatives as well, I now simply want to stay out of the psychiatric debate in general. This book is my final contribution.

In my twenties, I did my stint as a freelance journalist, and this book has been written with many of the techniques an undercover journalist might employ. I was determined to get to know the British mental health system from the inside out, and there were also times, particularly when I was on Dane Ward, that I much preferred the life of a psychiatric patient to actually going to work. One nurse actually accused me at one point of using Dane Ward "like a free hotel", and he was right!

Angels, Cleopatra and Psychosis

But at least I have researched my subject.

My basic objection to the current practice of psychiatry is that most psychiatrists believe and are taught to believe in a medical, biologically driven model of mental illness which they say they have proved to be true, but which I don't accept. And I am not the only sceptic. The psychiatrists Phil Thomas and Pat Bracken in *Post-Psychiatry* (OUP, 2005) also express their doubts, not least about the capitalist based relationship of psychiatry to the drugs companies, which both they and I object to. I also don't accept that schizophrenic symptoms necessarily constitute *dementia praecox* ("young dementia" as defined in the late 19th century by Emil Kraeplin), and neither am prepared to accept that manic depression is a proven biological illness either. There are all kinds of reasons why people can suffer from greatly fluctuating mood swings. Being unemployed one day and falling in love the next for example. There are some American psychiatrists who are now investigating manic depression on the grounds that its cause is a defective gene on the 11th chromosome, but what on earth does that actually *mean*? And what are their criteria for considering a gene to be defective? Why don't they just call it *different*? We live in a diverse world!

Kay Redfield Jamison, however, fascinates me both as a woman diagnosed with manic depression herself, and as one of the world's leading psychiatrists. Her autobiography *An Unquiet Mind* is well worth reading, and her book *Touched With Fire: Manic Depressive Illness And The Artistic Temperament* is a magnificent study of artists and art in itself, never mind its particular medical bent. For those wanting to know more, *Madness And Modernism* by Louis A. Sass is a comprehensive study of modern art's relationship to schizophrenia in particular, although I think it relies on the efficacy of the medical model too much. Further, the Manchester psychologist Richard Bentall's recent *Madness Explained* is comprehensive on current theory and medications, although I think the title is very arrogant! Second to last, *Psychiatric Drugs Explained* (2002) by David Healy is perhaps the best modern starting point. But the most informative and interesting book I have read on madness and its treatment is Phillippe Pinel's *A Treatise On Insanity* (1806). Pinel was a psychiatrist working at the Parisian asylums of Bîcetre (for men) and La Salpetiére (for women), and he was also working without the use of any psychiatric drugs, since none at that time had been invented. His solutions to his case studies are both highly imaginative and humane. *Vive la revolution!*

Now for my own thoughts based on my own experience as psychiatric laboratory guinea pig. I'm not quite sure how many drugs I have been on now, but the list goes something like Haloperidol, Largactil, Clopixol, Lithium (co-ordination problems), Clozaril (on which I was stable but it eventually started destroying my white blood cell immune system with a disease called neutropena), Olanzapine (rapid weight gain), sodium valproate (brand name Epilim) and aripiprazole (brand name Abilify). Only the last two have proved benign, and at doses so mild you could well argue as to whether they are effective at all. What I do know is that psychiatric drugs can frequently be a cause of mental disability in themselves. Risperdal Consta and Clopixol depot injections, in particular, make you comatose, you walk round like a zombie, and you are impotent as well. Why they are used by psychiatrists I just don't know! The side effects are far worse than the supposed disease.

Further, I am against the use of virtually all anti-psychotics, unless it is a dire emergency when the patient is becoming violent. I stand firm with *Asylum* magazine against the psychiatric assault of being pinned to the floor by six different nurses and being forcibly injected, and it has happened to me. Not only is it personally degrading, I consider it to be a fundamental human rights abuse.

As to the subject of angels I have only this to say. I have met four. Billy Graham says he has never met one, but his book *Angels: God's Secret Agents* is a useful study of angels' biblical significance, as is the far more recent *Angels* by Jane Williams (2006). Further, Hope Price's book *Angels* documents contemporary accounts of angelic visions and meetings, so I am not the only one to have gone through such experiences. Also, always remember that angelic language continues to be powerful in the popular song for instance – I think here of the work of Robbie Williams or Andrea Corr (solo or otherwise). Angels are integral to our cultural memory and perception of ourselves. As Annie Lennox once sang, "there must be an angel playing with my heart".

I don't think artists and scientists will ever agree on what constitutes proof of an events occurrence, but to the medical sceptic who dismisses my angelic meetings as psychotic I would say this. Firstly, in terms of hypomanic criteria, many creative people prefer to live slightly high lives (although I used to, I don't any more), and this should not be taken as a sign of illness. Secondly, as I understand it, virtually all anti-psychotic medications work by reducing the chemical dopamine production in the brain, and it is clear to me having been on many anti-psychotics that high levels of dopamine production in the brain are actually crucial to human creativity. I could go further and argue that you are only receptive to angelic experience when your dopamine levels are very high in the first place, but I can't prove it. I am however sure that the dopamine level reducing effects of anti-psychotics I have been forced to take against my will are partly why *The Minotaur* has been so difficult and taken such a long time to write, for example. Seven years to write it? It should have taken three.

Ultimately, you either believe in the existence of spirits and angels or you do not, according to your own personal experience. To perhaps the ultimate question of this book, "was I psychotic when I was visited by the angel Jana?" I would answer with two more questions rather central to our entire culture, and ones I have pondered many times. "Was the Virgin Mary psychotic when she was visited by the Archangel Gabriel?". And "how much dopamine did she have rushing round her brain when that happened?".

Angels, Cleopatra and Psychosis

Lightning Source UK Ltd.
Milton Keynes UK
UKOW02f1813081116
287183UK00001B/13/P